Drug Prescribing in Renal Failure

Dosing Guidelines for Adults

Third Edition

Also Available from the American College of Physicians

American College of Physicians Home Care Guide: Cancer
Clinical Practice Guidelines
Common Diagnostic Tests: Use and Interpretation—
    Second Edition
Common Screening Tests
Diagnostic Strategies for Common Medical Problems
Guide for Adult Immunization—Third Edition
Software for Internists

Publications from the *British Medical Journal* are now distributed in North America by the American College of Physicians.

Publications catalogue and ordering information for American College of Physicians and *British Medical Journal* publications are available from:

Customer Service
American College of Physicians
Independence Mall West
Sixth Street at Race
Philadelphia, PA 19106-1572
(215) 351-2600
(800) 523-1546

Drug Prescribing in Renal Failure

Dosing Guidelines for Adults

Third Edition

William M. Bennett
George R. Aronoff
Thomas A. Golper
Gail Morrison
D. Craig Brater
Irwin Singer

Published by the American College of Physicians
Philadelphia, Pennsylvania

Third Edition

Printed in the United States of America

Library of Congress Cataloging-in-Publication Data

Drug prescribing in renal failure : dosing guidelines for adults /
    William M. Bennett . . . [et al.]. — 3rd ed.
        159 pp.   cm.
        Includes bibliographical references and index.
        ISBN 0-943126-29-0 : $23.00 ($19.00 to ACP members)
        1. Chronic renal failure—Complications. 2. Drugs—Prescribing—
    Tables. 3. Drugs—Metabolism—Tables.   I. Bennett, William M.,
    1938–   .
        [DNLM: 1. Drugs—administration & dosage—tables. 2. Kidney
    Diseases—drug therapy—tables.   QV 16 D794 1994]
    RC918.R4D7   1994
    616.6' 1061—dc20
    DNLM/DLC
    for Library of Congress   93-49372
                                                                      CIP

The authors and publisher have exerted every effort to ensure that drug selection and dosage set forth in this manual are in accord with current recommendations and practice at the time of publication. In view of ongoing research, occasional changes in government regulations, and the constant flow of information relating to drug therapy and drug reactions, the reader is urged to check the package insert for each drug for any change in indications and dosage and for added warnings and precautions. This care is particularly important when the recommended agent is a new or infrequently used drug.

AUTHORS

George R. Aronoff, MD, FACP
Professor of Medicine
Chief, Division of Nephrology
University of Louisville
Louisville, Kentucky

William M. Bennett, MD, FACP
Professor of Medicine and Pharmacology
Head, Division of Nephrology and Hypertension
Oregon Health Sciences University
Portland, Oregon

D. Craig Brater, MD, FACP
Chairman, Department of Medicine
Indiana University School of Medicine
Indianapolis, Indiana

Thomas A. Golper, MD, FACP
Director of Dialysis-Related Services
Kidney Disease Program
University of Louisville
Louisville, Kentucky

Gail Morrison, MD, FACP
Associate Professor of Medicine
Associate Chairman, Department of Medicine
Hospital of the University of Pennsylvania
Associate Dean, Clinical Curriculum
University of Pennsylvania School of Medicine
Philadelphia, Pennsylvania

Irwin Singer, MD, FACP
Chief, Riviera Beach Outpatient Clinic
Miami Veterans Affairs Medical Center
Clinical Professor of Medicine
University of Miami School of Medicine
Miami, Florida

Contents

Introduction

Uremia affects every organ system and every aspect of drug disposition by the body. Because the kidney is the major regulator of the internal fluid environment, the physiologic changes associated with renal disease have pronounced effects on the pharmacology of many drugs. Clinicians must have a basic understanding of the biochemical and physiologic effects of drugs in patients with renal disease.

Bioavailability

The amount and appearance kinetics of a drug in the central circulation compared to intravenous dosing of the drug define its bioavailability (1). Drugs given intravenously enter the central circulation directly and generally have a rapid onset of action. Drugs given by other routes must first traverse a series of membranes and may need to pass through important organs of elimination before entering the systemic circulation. Only a fraction of the administered dose may reach the circulation and become available at the site of drug action.

Gastrointestinal absorption of drugs may decrease in patients with uremia. Gastrointestinal symptoms are common in uremia, but there is little specific information about bowel function in patients with renal failure. The gastric alkalinizing effect of salivary urea converted to ammonia by urease or by the use of histamine H_2-receptor antagonists may decrease the absorption of drugs that are best absorbed in an acidic environment (2). This effect is particularly important for patients receiving oral iron supplements that require conversion by acid from ferrous to ferric forms for absorption. The ingestion of milk or other sources of multivalent cations, such as aluminum-containing antacids, may decrease drug absorption by chelation and the formation of nonabsorbable complexes (3). In addition, uremic patients have decreased small bowel absorptive function (4).

First-pass hepatic metabolism may be altered in patients with uremia. Decreased biotransformation may lead to increased amounts of active drug in the systemic circulation and enhanced bioavailability of some drugs. Conversely, impaired plasma protein binding allows more free drug to be available at the site of hepatic metabolism, increasing the amount of drug removed during the hepatic first pass. The interactions of absorption and first-pass hepatic metabolism are complex. It is therefore not surprising that drug bioavailability varies more in patients with renal impairment than in patients with normal renal function.

Distribution

After administration, a drug disperses through the body at a given rate. At equilibrium, the apparent volume of distribution is the ratio of the amount of drug in the body to its plasma concentration. This ratio does not refer to a specific anatomic space but does provide an estimate for the initial dose of a drug needed to reach a therapeutic plasma concentration. Highly protein-bound agents, or those that are water soluble, tend to be restricted to the extracellular fluid space and have small volumes of distribution. On the other hand, drugs that are highly lipid soluble penetrate body tissues and exhibit large distribution volumes.

Renal insufficiency frequently alters drug distribution volume. Edema and ascites may increase the apparent volume of distribution of highly water-soluble or protein-bound drugs. Usual doses given to patients with edema may result in inadequate, low plasma levels. Conversely, dehydration or muscle wasting usually decreases the apparent volume of distribution of water-soluble drugs. In these cases, usual doses may result in unexpectedly high plasma concentrations.

The alteration of plasma protein binding in patients with renal insufficiency has an important effect on the volume of distribution of a drug, the quantity of free drug available for action, and the degree to which the agent can be excreted by the liver or kidneys. Protein-bound drugs attach reversibly either to albumin or glycoprotein in plasma. Organic acids often bind to a single site, whereas organic bases probably have several sites of attachment (5). The binding of many acidic drugs is decreased in renal failure. Binding of organic bases, on the other hand, is less affected by uremia (5).

Reduced plasma protein binding in uremic patients has been attributed to a combination of decreased serum albumin concentration and reduction in albumin affinity for the drug. Affinity may be influenced by either uremia-induced changes in the structural orientation of the albumin molecule or accumulation of endogenous inhibitors of protein binding that compete with drugs for their binding sites.

The therapeutic consequences of impaired plasma protein binding in uremia are important because the unbound fraction of several acidic drugs, such as salicylate and phenytoin, may be substantially increased. Serious toxicity could occur if the total plasma concentration were pushed into the therapeutic range by increasing the dose. For such drugs, total and unbound plasma concentrations should be measured.

Predicting the clinical consequences of altered protein binding in uremia is difficult. Although decreased binding results in more free drug being available at the site of drug action or toxicity, the distribution volume may be increased, producing lower plasma concentrations after a given dose. Because more unbound drug is available for metabolism and excretion, the half-life of the drug in the body may be decreased.

Metabolism

Renal failure substantially affects drug biotransformation. Reduction and hydrolysis reactions are generally slowed. Glucuronidation, sulfated conjugation, and microsomal oxidation usually occur at normal rates in patients with uremia (6).

Many active or toxic drug metabolites depend on renal function for elimination. The high incidence of adverse drug reactions seen in patients with renal failure may be explained in part by the accumulation of active metabolites (7).

Renal Excretion

Renal excretion of drugs depends on glomerular filtration and renal tubular secretion and reabsorption. Glomerular elimination of drugs also depends on the molecular size and protein-binding capacity of the agent. Although protein binding decreases the filtration of drugs, it may increase the amount the renal tubule secretes. When glomerular filtration is impaired by renal disease, the clearance of drugs eliminated primarily by this mechanism is decreased, and the plasma half-life of the drugs is prolonged.

Although we do not clinically measure tubular function, the secretion of drugs eliminated by active transport systems in the renal tubule is also affected in patients with renal disease. As the rate of creatinine clearance decreases, drugs dependent on renal tubular secretion for elimination are excreted more slowly. Furthermore, because the proximal tubular secretion of some agents is carrier mediated and capacity limited, concurrent use of several drugs eliminated by renal tubular secretion may saturate the transport system.

Pharmacokinetics

Pharmacokinetics deals with the time courses of drugs in the body and the construction of models to explain the absorption, distribution, metabolism, and excretion of drugs and their metabolites (1). After administration of the drug, an initial high plasma concentration is followed by a rapid decrease in the drug level. This decrease occurs as the drug is distributed from the plasma into the extravascular space. Concurrent with and after the distribution phase, the drug is eliminated at a slower rate. During the elimination phase, drug concentrations in plasma are in equilibrium with concentrations in body tissues.

Useful pharmacokinetic parameters can be developed using graphs of plasma drug concentrations after a dose is given. The rate and amount of drug absorption, the extent of distribution, and the rate of elimination are measured. By comparing pharmacokinetic data from patients with normal renal function to data from patients with renal insufficiency, rational drug dosimetry can be determined for patients with impaired renal function. The tables in this guide use specific pharmacokinetic information; however, for many drugs where data were inadequate or conflicting, the recommendations are based on the authors' judgments.

Dosimetry in Renal Disease

A rational approach to drug dosing in patients with renal impairment begins with a thorough history and physical examination. Particularly important is the history of previous drug allergy or toxicity, the use of concurrently prescribed or non-prescription medications, and the ingestion of alcohol or other recreational drugs. Physical assessment should include estimating the extracellular fluid volume because the presence of edema, ascites, or dehydration alters drug dose. Body weight and height need to be measured. For obese patients, the ideal body weight should be calculated, and drug doses should be estimated accordingly. Evidence of impaired excretory organ function should be sought. Signs of chronic liver disease are a clue that drug dose may need to be severely altered.

A specific diagnosis should be established before drug therapy is initiated. Patients with renal failure receive many concurrent medications, often without specific indications; therefore medication lists should be reviewed frequently. Many adverse drug effects could be avoided if fewer agents were used and potential drug interactions recognized.

Renal Function

When the necessity for drug therapy has been established, renal function should be measured. Because the rate of elimination of drugs excreted by the kidneys is proportional to the glomerular filtration rate, the serum creatinine or creatinine clearance should be used to estimate renal function. The equation of Cockroft and Gault (8) can be used to estimate the creatinine clearance as shown in the formula:

$$\text{Creatinine clearance} = \frac{(140 - \text{age}) \times \text{ideal body weight in kg}}{72 \times \text{serum creatinine in mg/dL}} \times 0.85 \text{ (for women)}$$

Ideal body weight for men = 50.0 kg + 2.3 kg per inch over 5 feet tall
Ideal body weight for women = 45.5 kg + 2.3 kg per inch over 5 feet tall

Estimating the glomerular filtration rate from the serum creatinine level assumes that renal function is stable and that the serum creatinine measurement is constant. With changing renal function, the serum creatinine level will no longer reflect the true clearance rate; creatinine clearance should be measured with a timed urine collection using the midpoint value. If oliguria is present, the creatinine clearance should be estimated at less than 10 mL/min.

The serum creatinine is a function of muscle mass as well as glomerular filtration rate. Serum creatinine measurements within the "normal" range are often erroneously used to establish the presence of "normal" renal function. Such an assumption could cause serious overdose and toxic drug accumulation in elderly or debilitated patients with diminished muscle mass.

Acute Renal Failure

The drug dosing guidelines in this book are mostly derived from studies done on patients with stable, chronic renal insufficiency. However, these recommendations are often extrapolated to seriously ill patients with acutely decreased renal function. Studies have shown that pharmacokinetic characteristics in patients with acute renal failure may differ from those measured in patients with chronic renal failure (9). Specifically, the nonrenal clearance of drugs decreases with the duration of renal failure. The preservation of nonrenal clearance observed early in the course of acute renal failure suggests that drug dosing schemes extrapolated from persons with stable chronic renal failure could possibly result in ineffectively low drug concentrations. Individualized pharmacokinetic dosing for patients with acute renal failure is essential early in the course of the patient's therapy.

Initial Dose

If the physical examination suggests that the extracellular fluid volume is normal, the initial drug dose for a patient with renal failure is the same as that for a patient with normal renal function. However, if substantial edema or ascites is present, a larger initial dose may be necessary. Conversely, dehydrated or severely debilitated patients may require smaller initial doses. The purpose of the initial, or loading, dose is to produce rapidly a therapeutic plasma drug concentration. Subsequent doses may need to be decreased to maintain therapeutic levels below the toxic range.

When a loading dose is given, levels within the therapeutic range are rapidly achieved. If no loading dose is prescribed, three to four half-lives of the drug will pass before the plasma levels are at steady state. A loading dose should always be considered when the half-life of a drug is particularly long in a patient with renal failure or when rapid attainment of therapeutic plasma levels is critical.

Maintenance Dose

After the initial drug dose, subsequent doses may need modification in patients with diminished renal function. After renal function has been measured and the drug dose for patients with normal renal function has been determined, the dose appropriate for patients with impaired renal function can be calculated. Guidelines for doses in patients with normal and impaired renal function are provided in the tables.

DRUG REMOVAL BY EXTRACORPOREAL TECHNIQUES

The effects of hemodialysis, peritoneal dialysis, and continuous arteriovenous or venovenous hemofiltration on drug elimination are difficult to predict. Factors affecting drug removal include molecular weight, lipid solubility, the chemistry and surface area of the dialysis membrane, blood and dialysate flow rates, drug protein binding, and red cell partitioning. During dialysis, intermittent changes in drug clearance disrupt the drug concentration equilibrium between the central and peripheral compartments. Redistribution from the deeper compartments into the vascular space results in a rebound of plasma drug concentrations after the dialysis treatment.

New techniques of extracorporeal circulation for the treatment of renal failure include continuous arteriovenous hemofiltration and continuous venovenous hemofiltration. These techniques use convective blood purification and continuous hemofiltration dialysis, which adds a diffusive component. Clearances of low-molecular-weight drugs are greater at higher dialysate flow rates because the removal of these compounds is substantially influenced by diffusion. Conversely, the clearance of high-molecular-weight compounds depends primarily on convection. Some compounds may even bind to some of the membranes used for hemofiltration.

Therapeutic Drug Monitoring

Clinical application of pharmacokinetic principles to individualize dosage regimens is called therapeutic drug monitoring. Recently developed sensitive and specific assays for plasma drug concentrations and inexpensive computer hardware and software are alternatives to drug dosing by trial and error. Appropriate pharmacokinetic application of drug level measurements can improve patient care at a decreased cost (10-12).

Measurement of plasma drug concentrations may help in assessing a particular drug dosing regimen when the relation between drug levels and efficacy or toxicity has been established. These measurements are particularly important for drugs with a narrow range between therapeutic and toxic levels and for drugs whose pharmacologic effects are not readily measured. Plasma level monitoring, however, has little value for drugs with an effect that is easily measured or irreversible. For example, the efficacy of antihypertensive medications parallels plasma drug concentrations but can be easily determined by monitoring blood pressure and heart rate.

Generally, three or four doses of the drug should be given before plasma levels are measured to ensure that steady-state concentrations have been established. For some drugs, both maximum and minimum concentrations are relevant. Peak levels are most meaningful when measured after rapid drug distribution has occurred. For example, aminoglycoside peak concentrations are usually measured 30 minutes after the infusion. Minimum plasma drug concentrations should be measured immediately before the next dose is given. Trough levels are more reliable measurements of drug elimination and reflect more closely potential drug accumulation in patients with renal failure.

Many institutions offer formal dosing services. Although often based in the pharmacy, these services should be multidisciplinary, including the primary physician and subspecialty consultants. Based on the patient's clinical state, concurrent medications, blood level pharmacokinetics, and response to therapy, consultants provide advice on drug dose, interval, route of administration, and timing of plasma levels. Final recommendations often include literature references, adverse drug effects, and potential drug interactions (12).

Adverse Drug Reactions

Despite careful consideration of uremia-induced changes in drug disposition, adverse drug responses remain common in patients with impaired renal function (13, 14). Some toxicity can be eliminated by avoiding drugs known to cause adverse events as a result of direct toxicity of the drug or its metabolites, poor efficacy of the drug in decreased renal function, or production of an increased metabolic load that diseased kidneys cannot excrete.

Knowing a drug's potential for direct renal toxicity is particularly important for patients with reduced renal function. Even a mild renal injury in a patient with diminished renal reserve can be catastrophic. Drugs may precipitate direct renal tubule toxicity, obstructive uropathy, glomerulonephritis, interstitial nephritis, and disturbances of sodium and water and acid-base balance. The accumulation of active or toxic metabolites may lead to unexpected drug reactions. Acute onset of any unexplained symptoms should alert clinicians to a possible adverse drug effect.

Patients with renal failure are heterogeneous, and their responses to drug therapy are variable. Dosage nomograms, dosage tables, and computer-assisted dosing recommendations should not be used as a fixed approach but as an initial attempt to arrive at an effective dose regime. The authors have included in the tables the dose of most drugs used for patients with normal renal function. These doses vary with the specific needs of each patient and include appropriate adjustment for patients with renal failure. In addition, specific supplementary doses for patients having hemodialysis, continuous ambulatory peritoneal dialysis, and continuous arteriovenous or venovenous hemofiltration are provided. Physicians using sound clinical judgment in caring for patients with renal disease evaluate each situation, choose a drug regimen based on all factors, and continually reevaluate response to therapy.

Pharmacokinetic studies have led to the development of inclusive nomograms and tables of drug disposition and dosimetry for patients with renal impairment. The tables in this book contain dose recommendations based on the most current information available; that information is liberally quoted (15-19).

References

1. **Wagner JG.** Fundamentals of Clinical Pharmacokinetics. Hamilton, Illinois: Drug Intelligence Publications, Inc.; 1975:337-58.
2. **Anderson RJ, Gambertoglio JG, Schrier RW.** Clinical Use of Drugs in Renal Failure. Springfield, Illinois: Charles C Thomas; 1976.
3. **Hurwitz A.** Antacid therapy and drug kinetics. Clin Pharmacokinet. 1977;2:269-80.
4. **Craig R, Murphy T, Gibson TP.** Kinetic analysis of D-xylose absorption in normal subjects and in patients with chronic renal insufficiency. J Lab Clin Med. 1983;101:496-506.
5. **Reidenberg MM.** The binding of drugs to plasma proteins and the interpretation of measurements of plasma concentration of drugs in patients with poor renal function. Am J Med. 1977;62:466-70.
6. **Reidenberg MM.** The biotransformation of drugs in renal failure. Am J Med. 1977;62:482-5.
7. **Verbeeck RK, Branch RA, Wilkinson GR.** Drug metabolites in renal failure: pharmacokinetic and clinical implications. Clin Pharmacokinet. 1981;6:329-45.

8. **Cockroft DW, Gault MH.** Prediction of creatinine clearance from serum creatinine. Nephron. 1976;16:31-41.

9. **Macias WL, Mueller BA, Scarim SK.** Vancomycin pharmacokinetics in acute renal failure: preservation of nonrenal clearance. Clin Phamacol Ther. 1991;50:688-94.

10. **Bollish SJ, Kelly WN, Miller DE, Timmons RG.** Establishing an aminoglycoside pharmacokinetic monitoring service in a community hospital. Am J Hosp Pharm. 1981;38:73-6.

11. **Elenbaas RM, Payne VW, Bauman JL.** Influence of clinical pharmacist consultations on the use of drug blood level tests. Am J Hosp Pharm. 1980;37:61-4.

12. **Aronoff GR, Abel SR.** Principles of administering drugs to patients with renal failure. In: Brenner BM, Stein JH, eds. Contemporary Issues in Nephrology. New York: Churchill-Livingstone; 1986:1-19.

13. **Jick H.** Adverse drug effects in relation to renal function. Am J Med. 1977;62:514-7.

14. **Smith JW, Seidl LG, Cluff LE.** Studies on the epidemiology of adverse drug reaction. V. Clinical factors influencing susceptibility. Ann Intern Med. 1966;65:629-40.

15. **Fillastre JP, Singlas E.** Pharmacokinetics of newer drugs in patients with renal impairment. Clin Pharmacokinet. 1991;20:293-310.

16. **Swan SK, Bennett WM.** Drug dosing guidelines in patients with renal failure. West J Med. 1992;156:633-8.

17. **Bryan CS, Stone WJ.** Antimicrobial dosage in renal failure: a unifying nomogram. Clin Nephrol. 1977;7:81-4.

18. **Tozer TN.** Nomogram for modification of dosage regimens in patients with chronic renal function impairment. J Pharmacokinet Biopharm. 1974;2:13-28.

19. **Bennett WM, Aronoff GR, Golper TA, Morrison G, Singer I, Brater DC.** Drug Prescribing in Renal Failure: Dosing Guidelines for Adults. Philadelphia: American College of Physicians; 1991.

Use of the Tables

Drugs in this book are listed by generic name, in alphabetical order, under subdivisions based on similarity of structure and pharmacologic action. For example, penicillins, cephalosporins, and aminoglycosides are grouped together as antibiotics.

Toxicity and Notes

Nephrotoxicity or systemic adverse effects and information specifically related to patients with renal disease are listed directly under the generic drug name. Remarks common to all members of a class or group of drugs are listed under the name of the drug class and generally apply to each drug in the group.

Route of Excretion

The second column lists the percentage of total drug excreted unchanged in the urine for patients with normal renal function. For some drugs, the second column gives the major route of elimination or metabolism. Drugs extensively metabolized by the liver or extracted during initial circulation through the liver after gastrointestinal absorption have complex pharmacokinetics. For these drugs, the half-life given is for the disappearance of active drug after it has reached the general circulation. In patients with hepatic dysfunction, the percentage of an administered dose metabolized by the "first pass" effect may be reduced. For the tables, it is assumed liver function is normal and that other drugs that alter hepatic metabolism are not being given.

Pharmacokinetic Variables

Dosage adjustments for renal failure depend on knowledge of normal drug disposition. Pharmacokinetic variables in normal subjects are given in the tables. These variables include the major route of drug elimination by either excretion or metabolism, the plasma or biological half-life for patients with normal renal function or end-stage renal disease, the extent of drug binding to plasma proteins, and the apparent volume of distribution. The volume of distribution and half-life given should be considered in estimating blood levels after dosage, in finding the proper maintenance regimen, and in deciding the likelihood of drug removal by dialysis. As outlined above, the complex pharmacokinetics and variability of drug disposition in patients with renal failure cannot be adequately described by these simple parameters.

Dose for Normal Renal Function

After the column listing pharmacokinetic variables, drug doses sometimes given to patients with normal renal function are listed. These recommendations are meant only as a guide and do not imply efficacy of a listed dosage.

Dosage Adjustment for Renal Failure

A loading dose should be considered when the half-life of a drug is particularly long in patients with impaired renal function. When the physical examination suggests that the extracellular fluid volume is normal, the loading dose of a drug given to a patient with renal insufficiency is the same as the initial dose given to a patient with normal renal function. Initial doses for most drugs requiring loading are already known. However, the loading dose may be calculated using the following formula:

Loading dose = Vd (L/kg) × Wt (kg) × Cp (mg/L)

    Vd = volume of distribution of the drug
    Wt = patient's ideal body weight
    Cp = desired plasma drug level

If the patient has substantial edema or ascites, a somewhat larger loading dose may be required. Conversely, dehydrated or debilitated patients should receive smaller initial drug doses.

To adjust the maintenance dosage in patients with renal insufficiency, the intervals between individual doses can be lengthened (interval extension method), keeping the dose size normal. The calculated dose interval should be rounded off to create a convenient time schedule. This method is particularly useful for drugs with wide therapeutic ranges and long plasma half-lives in patients with renal impairment. Lengthening the interval will result in wide swings of the plasma drug concentrations from peak to trough levels. If the range between the therapeutic and toxic levels is too narrow, either toxic or subtherapeutic plasma concentrations may result.

Alternatively, the size of the individual doses can be reduced, keeping the interval between doses normal. Decreasing the individual doses reduces the difference between peak and trough plasma concentrations. This effect is important to note for drugs with narrow therapeutic ranges and short plasma half-lives in patients with renal impairment. Decreasing dose size is recommended for drugs in which a relatively constant blood level is desired. The reduced dose should be rounded off to a convenient value.

In the tables, the preferred method for dosage adjustment is included for each drug. Dose reduction is indicated by "D," and interval extension, by "I." After the recommended method for dosage adjustment, recommendations are given for levels of renal function as estimated by the glomerular filtration rate. For the dose-reduction method, the percentage of the usual dose to be given at the normal dose interval is shown. When the interval extension method is recommended, the number of hours between doses of normal size is given.

No controlled clinical trials have been done to establish the efficacy of the two methods for drug-dose alteration in patients with renal insufficiency. Prolonging the dose interval is often more convenient and less expensive. When the dose interval can safely be lengthened beyond 24 hours, extended parenteral therapy can be completed without prolonged hospitalization. In patients requiring chronic hemodialysis, many drugs need to be given only at the end of the dialysis treatment. Further, compliance with any drug regimen may be better when fewer doses can be taken at convenient times.

In practice, a combination of interval prolongation and dose-size reduction is often effective and convenient. The recommendations given for aminoglycosides are an attempt to combine these considerations by decreasing the individual aminoglycoside doses and increasing the dosage interval. These recommendations are shown by "D" and "I."

Dialysis Adjustment

The effect of standard clinical treatment on drug removal is shown for hemodialysis (Hemo), chronic ambulatory peritoneal dialysis (CAPD), and continuous arteriovenous or venovenous hemofiltration (CAVH). When known, specific recommendations for dose adjustment are given. Some drugs that have high dialysis clearance do not require supplemental doses after dialysis if the amount of drug removed is not sufficient, as would be the case if the volume of distribution is large. To ensure efficacy when information about dialysis loss is not available and to simplify dosimetry, maintenance doses of most drugs should be given after dialysis.

Peritonitis is a major complication of CAPD, and treatment usually involves intraperitoneal administration of antibiotics. For some drugs sophisticated pharmacokinetic studies are available, whereas for other drugs use is still based on empiric dosage recommendations. Drug absorption is generally excellent after intraperitoneal administration of common antibiotics. Factors favoring absorption include inflamed membranes and concentration gradients. For drugs such as aminoglycosides, cephalosporins, and penicillins, the drug levels in peritoneal fluid after intravenous or oral administration are inconsistent.

The following abbreviations are used in the tables:

BUN—blood urea nitrogen; Ca^{++}—factor IV calcium; CAPD—chronic ambulatory peritoneal dialysis; CAVH—continuous arteriovenous or venovenous hemofiltration; CNS—central nervous system; D—dosage reduction method; ESRD—end-stage renal disease; GFR—glomerular filtration rate; Hemo—hemodialysis; I—interval extension method; K^{+}—potassium; Mg^{++}—magnesium; Na^{+}—sodium; NSAIDs—nonsteroidal anti-inflammatory drugs; PO_4—phosphate radical; SIADH—syndrome of inappropriate secretion of antidiuretic hormone; T 1/2—biologic half life; UTI—urinary tract infection.

Antimicrobial Agents

Antimicrobial therapy in patients with renal disease begins with an attempt to isolate the causative organism. Often uremic patients with serious infections do not have elevated temperatures, and nonspecific symptoms of infection may be attributed to uremia or the effects of dialysis. Because patients with renal insufficiency are more likely to have adverse effects from antimicrobial therapy than are patients with normal renal function, culture documentation of bacterial infection is essential. When patients are seriously ill, antimicrobial therapy must be chosen empirically, but only after exhaustive attempts to isolate specific pathogens.

The choice of antimicrobial agents includes consideration of potential toxicity. The consequences of inadvertent drug or metabolite accumulation must be considered, and side effects rarely seen in patients with normal renal function may occur more frequently in patients with renal failure. For example, seizures from beta-lactam accumulation are rare in patients with sufficient kidney function to prevent drug accumulation but can occur in patients with renal impairment when large doses are given.

Mild nephrotoxicity in patients with renal insufficiency may result in overt uremia. A decrease in renal function of as much as 50% from aminoglycoside nephrotoxicity can go unnoticed in patients with normal baseline kidney function. A similar change in patients with creatinine clearance rates less than 20 mL/min might precipitate the need for dialysis.

Accumulation of metabolic waste products must also be considered in patients with impaired excretory capacity. The anti-anabolic effects of tetracyclines can cause an increase in the blood urea nitrogen. Drugs that increase metabolic load should be avoided.

Most antimicrobial agents are eliminated by the kidneys. For most of these drugs, detailed kinetic studies in patients with renal impairment have led to detailed dosing guidelines. However, the derived suggestions are appropriate for the "average" patient and are only a starting point for individualization of therapy.

Although some antimicrobial agents have a narrow therapeutic index, many are relatively nontoxic. These drugs show a great difference among their therapeutic and toxic plasma concentrations. Dose reduction that results in ineffectively low plasma concentrations is the greatest danger in prescribing these antimicrobial agents for patients with renal impairment. The aminoglycoside antibiotic agents have the narrowest therapeutic range of any of the antimicrobial drugs. These agents are eliminated almost exclusively by glomerular filtration, and accumulation can cause nephrotoxicity and ototoxicity. Precise dose reduction, drug-level monitoring, and careful repeated measurements of renal function are required in patients receiving aminoglycoside therapy.

To reach therapeutic plasma drug levels rapidly, the initial dose of antimicrobial agents for patients with impaired renal function should be the same as that for patients with normal renal function. If substantial edema or ascites is present, a larger initial dose may be necessary. Conversely, dehydrated or severely debilitated patients may require smaller initial doses.

No controlled clinical trials have compared the relative efficacy of modifying drug dose in renal insufficiency by decreasing the individual doses or by increasing the dose interval. When subsequent doses need to be decreased because of diminished renal function, for most antimicrobial agents the dose should be modified by prolonging the dose interval. Because the wide therapeutic range of most of these drugs allows for higher peak levels without toxicity and lower trough levels without loss of efficacy, the dose interval often may be extended to 24 hours or more. Extension of the dose interval is more convenient and less expensive; when the clinical situation permits, outpatient parenteral antimicrobial therapy may be given.

To eliminate the risk of ineffectively low plasma drug concentrations in seriously ill patients, we prefer not to extend the dose interval beyond 24 hours. In such patients a decrease in the individual doses combined with prolonging the dose interval maintains safe, therapeutic drug levels. This combined approach results in therapeutic efficacy, convenience, and cost savings.

Because there is often a direct relation between plasma levels and antimicrobial efficacy or toxicity, drug levels should be measured. Generally, three or four doses should be given before levels are measured to ensure that steady-state concentrations have been established. For some drugs, both maximum and minimum concentrations are relevant. Peak levels are most meaningful when measured after rapid drug distribution has occurred. Minimum plasma drug concentrations should be measured immediately before the next dose is to be given. These trough levels are more reliable measurements of elimination and reflect more closely potential drug accumulation in patients with renal failure. Drug level monitoring is particularly important in patients with unstable renal function.

Antimicrobial Agents

Drug, Toxicity Notes	Percent Excreted Unchanged	Half-Life (Normal/ ESRD)	Plasma Protein Binding	Volume of Distribution	Dose for Normal Renal Function	Adjustment for Renal Failure — Method	GFR, mL/min >50	10-50	<10	Supplement for Dialysis
	%	h	%	L/kg						

Antibacterial Antibiotics

Aminoglycoside Antibiotics

Nephrotoxic. Ototoxic. Toxicity worse when hyperbilirubinemic. Measure serum levels for efficacy and toxicity. Peritoneal absorption increases with presence of inflammation. Volume of distribution increases with edema, obesity, and ascites.

Drug, Toxicity Notes	Percent Excreted Unchanged (%)	Half-Life (Normal/ESRD) (h)	Plasma Protein Binding (%)	Volume of Distribution (L/kg)	Dose for Normal Renal Function	Method	>50	10-50	<10	Supplement for Dialysis
Amikacin	95	1.4-2.3/17-150	< 5	0.22-0.29	5 mg/kg q8h	D and I	60-90% q12h	30-70% q12-18h	20-30% q24-48h	Hemo: 2/3 normal dose after dialysis CAPD: 15-20 mg/L · d CAVH: Dose for GFR 10-50 and measure levels
Gentamicin	95	1.8/20-60	< 5	0.23-0.26	1-1.5 mg/kg q8h	D and I	60-90% q8-12h	30-70% q12h	20-30% q24-48h	Hemo: 2/3 normal dose after dialysis CAPD: 3-4 mg/L · d CAVH: Dose for GFR 10-50 and measure levels

Concurrent penicillins may result in subtherapeutic aminoglycoside levels.

Drug				Dose	Method	>50	10-50	<10	Supplement for dialysis
Kanamycin	50-90	1.8-5/40-96	< 5	0.19-0.23	5 mg/kg q8h	D and I	60-90% q8-12h	30-70% q12h	20-30% q24-48h	Hemo: 2/3 normal dose after dialysis CAPD: 15-20 mg/L · d CAVH: Dose for GFR 10-50 and measure levels
Netilmicin	95	1-3/35-72	< 5	0.16-0.30	5 mg/kg q8h	D and I	50-90% q8-12h	20-60% q12h	10-20% q24-48h	Hemo: 2/3 normal dose after dialysis CAPD: 3-4 mg/L · d CAVH: Dose for GFR 10-50 and measure levels

May be less ototoxic than other members of class.

Drug				Dose	Method	>50	10-50	<10	Supplement for dialysis
Streptomycin	70	2.5/100	35	0.26	1 g/d	I	q24h	q24-72h	q72-96h	Hemo: 1/2 normal dose after dialysis CAPD: 20-40 mg/L · d CAVH: Dose for GFR 10-50 and measure levels

May be less nephrotoxic than other members of class.

Drug				Dose	Method	>50	10-50	<10	Supplement for dialysis
Tobramycin	95	2.5/27-60	< 5	0.22-0.33	1-1.5 mg/kg q8h	D and I	60-90% q8-12h	30-70% q12h	20-30% q24-48h	Hemo: 2/3 normal dose after dialysis CAPD: 3-4 mg/L · d CAVH: Dose for GFR 10-50 and measure levels

Concurrent penicillins may result in subtherapeutic aminoglycoside levels.

For definitions of the abbreviations used in the tables, see page 14.

Antimicrobial Agents (Continued)

Drug, Toxicity Notes	Percent Excreted Unchanged	Half-Life (Normal/ ESRD)	Plasma Protein Binding	Volume of Distribution	Dose for Normal Renal Function	Adjustment for Renal Failure				Supplement for Dialysis
						Method	GFR, mL/min			
							>50	10-50	<10	
	%	h	%	L/kg						

Cephalosporin Antibiotics

Rare allergic interstitial nephritis. Absorbed well when given intraperitoneally. May cause bleeding from impaired prothrombin biosynthesis.

Drug	%	h	%	L/kg		Method	>50	10-50	<10	Supplement for Dialysis
Cefaclor	70	1/3	25	0.24-0.35	250-500 mg tid	D	100%	50-100%	50%	Hemo: 250 mg after dialysis CAPD: 250 mg q8-12h CAVH: Not applicable
Cefadroxil	70-90	1.4-22	20	0.31	0.5-1.0 g q12h	I	q12h	q12-24h	q24-48h	Hemo: 0.5-1.0 g after dialysis CAPD: 0.5 g/d CAVH: Not applicable
Cefamandole	50-100	1/6-11	75	0.16-0.25	0.5-1.0 g q4-8h	I	q6h	q6-8h	q12h	Hemo: 0.5-1.0 g after dialysis CAPD: 0.5-1.0 g q12h CAVH: Dose for GFR 10-50

						q8h	q12h	q24-48h	
Cefazolin	75-95	2/40-70	80	0.13-0.22	0.5-1.5 g q6h	I	q8h	q12h	q24-48h	Hemo: 0.5-1.0 g after dialysis CAPD: 0.5 g q12h CAVH: Dose for GFR 10-50
Cefepime	85	2.2/18	16	0.3	250-2000 mg q8h	I	q12h	q16-24h	q24-48h	Hemo: 1 g after dialysis CAPD: Dose for GFR < 10 CAVH: Not recommended
Cefixime	18-50	3.1/12	50	0.6-1.1	200 mg q12h	D	100%	75%	50%	Hemo: 300 mg after dialysis CAPD: 200 mg/d CAVH: Not recommended

400 mg/d to treat peritonitis.

Cefmenoxime	70	0.8-1.3/6-12	43-75	0.27-0.37	1 g q6h	D and I	1.0 g q8h	0.75 g q8h	0.75 g q12h	Hemo: 0.75 g after dialysis CAPD: 0.75 g q12h CAVH: Dose for GFR 10-50
Cefmetazole	85	1.2/21	75	0.18	2 g q6-12h	I	q16h	q24h	q48h	Hemo: Dose after dialysis CAPD: Dose for GFR < 10 CAVH: Dose for GFR 10-50

Probenecid doubles half-life.

Cefonicid	95	4/17-59	96	0.09-0.18	1 g/d	D and I	0.5 g/d	0.1-0.5 g/d	0.1 g/d	Hemo: None CAPD: None CAVH: None
Cefoperazone	20	1.6-2.5/2.9	90	0.14-0.20	1-2 g q12h	D	100%	100%	100%	Hemo: 1 g after dialysis CAPD: None CAVH: None

Displaced from protein by bilirubin. Reduce dose by 50% for jaundice.
May prolong prothrombin time.

For definitions of the abbreviations used in the tables, see page 14.

Antimicrobial Agents (Continued)

Drug, Toxicity Notes	Percent Excreted Unchanged %	Half-Life (Normal/ESRD) h	Plasma Protein Binding %	Volume of Distribution L/kg	Dose for Normal Renal Function	Method	GFR, mL/min >50	GFR, mL/min 10-50	GFR, mL/min <10	Supplement for Dialysis
Ceforanide	85	3/25	80	0.17	0.5-1.0 g q12h	I	q12h	q12-24h	q24-48h	Hemo: 0.5-1.0 g after dialysis CAPD: None CAVH: 1 g/d
Cefotaxime	60	1/15	37	0.15-0.55	1 g q6h	I	q6h	q8-12h	q24h	Hemo: 1 g after dialysis CAPD: 1 g/d CAVH: 1 g q12h
Cefotetan Active metabolite in ESRD. Reduce dose further for hepatic and renal failure.	75	3.5/13-25	85	0.15	1-2 g q12h	D	100%	50%	25%	Hemo: 1 g after dialysis CAPD: 1 g/d CAVH: 750 mg q12h
Cefoxitin	80	1/13-23	41-75	0.2	1-2 g q6-8h	I	q8h	q8-12h	q24-48h	Hemo: 1 g after dialysis CAPD: 1 g/d CAVH: Dose for GFR 10-50
Cefpodoxime May falsely increase serum creatinine by interference with assay.	30	2.5/26	26	0.6-1.2	200 mg q12h	I	q12h	q16h	q24-48h	Hemo: 200 mg after dialysis only CAPD: Dose for GFR < 10 CAVH: Not applicable

Drug	%	t½ (normal/ESRD)	%	Vd	Dose	D and I	q12h / 100% (>50)	q12-16h / 100% (10-50)	q24h / 100% (<10)	Dialysis
Cefprozil	65	1.7/6	40	0.65	500 mg q12h	D and I	250 mg q12h	250 mg q12-16h	250 mg q24h	Hemo: 250 mg after dialysis CAPD: Dose for GFR < 10 CAVH: Dose for GFR < 10
Ceftazidime	60-85	1.2/13-25	17	0.28-0.4	1-2 g q8h	I	q8-12h	q24-48h	q48h	Hemo: 1 g after dialysis CAPD: 0.5 g/d CAVH: Dose for GFR 10-50

Volume of distribution increases with infection.

Drug	%	t½	%	Vd	Dose	D and I	>50	10-50	<10	Dialysis
Ceftizoxime	57-100	1.4/35	28-50	0.26-0.42	1-2 g q8-12h	I	q8-12h	q12-24h	q24h	Hemo: 1 g after dialysis CAPD: 0.5-1.0 g/d CAVH: Dose for GFR 10-50
Ceftriaxone	30-65	7-9/12-24	90	0.12-0.18	0.2-1.0 g q12h	D	100%	100%	100%	Hemo: Dose after dialysis CAPD: 750 mg q12h CAVH: Dose for GFR 10-50

Monitor levels in dialysis patients.

Drug	%	t½	%	Vd	Dose	D and I	>50	10-50	<10	Dialysis
Cefuroxime axetil	90	1.2/17	35-50	0.13-1.8	250-500 mg q12h	D	100%	100%	100%	Hemo: Dose after dialysis CAPD: Dose for GFR < 10 CAVH: Not applicable

Malabsorbed in presence of H_2 blockers. Absorbed better with food.

Drug	%	t½	%	Vd	Dose	D and I	>50	10-50	<10	Dialysis
Cefuroxime sodium	90	1.2/17	33	0.13-1.8	0.75-1.5 g q8h	I	q8h	q8-12h	q24h	Hemo: Dose after dialysis CAPD: Dose for GFR < 10 CAVH: 1 g q12h
Cephalexin	98	0.7/16	20	0.35	250-500 mg q6h	I	q8h	q12h	q12h	Hemo: Dose after dialysis CAPD: Dose for GFR < 10 CAVH: Not applicable

For definitions of the abbreviations used in the tables, see page 14.

Antimicrobial Agents (Continued)

Drug, Toxicity Notes	Percent Excreted Unchanged	Half-Life (Normal/ESRD)	Plasma Protein Binding	Volume of Distribution	Dose for Normal Renal Function	Adjustment for Renal Failure GFR, mL/min				Supplement for Dialysis
						Method	>50	10-50	<10	
	%	h	%	L/kg						
Cephalothin	60-90	0.5-1/3-18	65	0.26	0.5-2.0 g q6h	I	q6h	q6-8h	q12h	Hemo: Dose after dialysis CAPD: 1 g q12h CAVH: 1 g q8h
Cephapirin	60	0.4/2.5	45-60	0.22	0.5-2.0 g q6h	I	q6h	q6-8h	q12h	Hemo: Dose after dialysis CAPD: 1 g q12h CAVH: 1 g q8h
Cephradine	100	0.7-1.3/6-15	10	0.25-0.46	0.25-2.0 g q6h	D	100%	50%	25%	Hemo: Dose after dialysis CAPD: Dose for GFR < 10 CAVH: Not applicable
Moxalactam (Latamoxef) Sodium, 3.8 mEq/g. Monitor prothrombin time or give vitamin K. Platelet dysfunction at high doses.	61-79	2.3/18-23	35-59	0.18-0.40	1-2 g q8-12h	I	q8-12h	q12-24h	q24-48h	Hemo: Dose after dialysis CAPD: Dose for GFR < 10 CAVH: Dose for GFR 10-50

Miscellaneous Antibacterial Antibiotics

Drug, Toxicity Notes	Percent Excreted Unchanged	Half-Life (Normal/ESRD)	Plasma Protein Binding	Volume of Distribution	Dose for Normal Renal Function	Method	>50	10-50	<10	Supplement for Dialysis
Azithromycin ESRD dosing recommendations based on extrapolation as no data are yet available.	6-12	10-60/?	8-50	18	250-500 mg/d	D	100%	100%	100%	Hemo: None CAPD: None CAVH: None

Drug							>50	10–50	<10	
Aztreonam	75	1.7-2.9/6-8	55	0.1-2.0	1-2 g q8-12h	D	100%	50-75%	25%	Hemo: 0.5 g after dialysis CAPD: Dose for GFR < 10 CAVH: Dose for GFR 10-50
Chloramphenicol	10	1.6-3.3/3-7	45-60	0.5-1.0	12.5 mg/kg q6h	D	100%	100%	100%	Hemo: None CAPD: None CAVH: None
Cilastin	60	1/12	44	0.22	With imipenem	D	100%	50%	Avoid	Hemo: Avoid CAPD: Avoid CAVH: Avoid

Unnecessary in renal failure.

| Clarithromycin | 15 | 2.3-6/? | 70 | 2-4 | 500-1000 mg q12h | D | 100% | 75% | 50-75% | Hemo: Dose after dialysis
CAPD: None
CAVH: None |

ESRD dosing recommendations based on extrapolation as no data are yet available.

| Clavulanic acid | 40 | 1/3-4 | 30 | 0.3 | 100 mg q4-6h | D | 100% | 100% | 50-75% | Hemo: Dose after dialysis
CAPD: Dose for GFR < 10
CAVH: Dose for GFR 10-50 |

Only used in fixed combination with ticarcillin or amoxicillin.

| Clindamycin | 10 | 2-4/3-5 | 60-95 | 0.6-1.2 | 150-300 mg q6h | D | 100% | 100% | 100% | Hemo: None
CAPD: None
CAVH: None |
| Erythromycin | 15 | 1.4/5-6 | 60-95 | 0.78 | 250-500 mg q6-12h | D | 100% | 100% | 50-75% | Hemo: None
CAPD: None
CAVH: None |

Ototoxicity with high doses in ESRD. Volume of distribution increases in ESRD.

| Imipenem | 20-70 | 1/4 | 13-21 | 0.17-0.3 | 0.25-1.0 g q6h | D | 100% | 50% | 25% | Hemo: Dose after dialysis
CAPD: Dose for GFR < 10
CAVH: Dose for GFR 10-50 |

Seizures in ESRD. Nonrenal clearance in acute renal failure is less than in chronic renal failure. Administered with cilastin to prevent nephrotoxicity of renal metabolite.

For definitions of the abbreviations used in the tables, see page 14.

25

Antimicrobial Agents (Continued)

Drug, Toxicity Notes	Percent Excreted Unchanged %	Half-Life (Normal/ESRD) h	Plasma Protein Binding %	Volume of Distribution L/kg	Dose for Normal Renal Function	Adjustment for Renal Failure Method	GFR, mL/min >50	10-50	<10	Supplement for Dialysis
Lincomycin	10-15	4-5/10-20	70-80	0.31-0.6	0.5 g q6h	I	q6h	q6-12h	q12-24h	Hemo: None CAPD: None CAVH: Not applicable
Meropenem	65	1.1/6-8	Low	0.35	500-1000 mg q6h	D and I	500 mg q6h	250-500 mg q12h	250-500 mg q24h	Hemo: Dose after dialysis CAPD: Dose for GFR < 10 CAVH: Dose for GFR 10-50
Methenamine mandelate	High	4/Unknown	Unknown	Unknown	1.0 g q6h	D	100%	Avoid	Avoid	Hemo: Not applicable CAPD: Not applicable CAVH: Not applicable
Metronidazole	20	6-14/7-21	20	0.25-0.85	7.5 mg/kg q6h	D	100%	100%	50%	Hemo: Dose after dialysis CAPD: Dose for GFR < 10 CAVH: Dose for GFR 10-50
Metabolites accumulate. Rare drug-induced lupus.										
Nitrofurantoin	30-40	0.5/1	20-60	0.3-0.7	50-100 mg q6h	D	100%	Avoid	Avoid	Hemo: Not applicable CAPD: Not applicable CAVH: Not applicable
Spectinomycin	35-90	1.6/16-29	5-20	0.25	2-4 g once	D	100%	100%	100%	Hemo: None CAPD: None CAVH: None

Drug				Normal Dose	Method	>50	10-50	<10	Dialysis
Sulbactam	50-80	1/10-21	30	0.25-0.50	0.75-1.5 g q6-8h	I	q6-8h	q12-24h	q24-48h	Hemo: Dose after dialysis; CAPD: 0.75-1.5 g/d; CAVH: 750 mg q12h
Beta lactamase inhibitor combined with ampicillin.									
Sulfamethoxazole	70	10/20-50	50	0.28-0.38	1.0 g q8h	I	q12h	q18h	q24h	Hemo: 1 g after dialysis; CAPD: 1 g/d; CAVH: Dose for GFR 10-50
Recommendation as single agent. Protein binding decreased in ESRD. Use normal dosing for UTI in ESRD.									
Sulfisoxazole	70	3-7/6-12	85	0.14-0.28	1-2 g q6h	I	q6h	q8-12h	q12-24h	Hemo: 2 g after dialysis; CAPD: 3 g/d; CAVH: Not applicable
Protein binding decreased in ESRD. Use normal dosing for UTI in ESRD.									
Tazobactam	65	1/7	22	0.21	1.5-2.25 g/d	D	100%	75%	50%	Hemo: 1/3 dose after dialysis; CAPD: Dose for GFR < 10; CAVH: Dose for GFR 10-50
Combined with pipercillin and dose adjustments determined by pipercillin.									
Teicoplanin	40-60	33-190/62-230	60-90	0.5-1.2	6 mg/kg · d	I	q24h	q48h	q72h	Hemo: Dose for GFR < 10; CAPD: Dose for GFR < 10; CAVH: Dose for GFR 10-50
Trimethoprim	40-70	9-13/20-49	30-70	1-2.2	100-200 mg q12h	I	q12h	q18h	q24h	Hemo: Dose after dialysis; CAPD: q24h; CAVH: q18h
Vancomycin	90-100	6-8/200-250	10-50	0.47-1.1	500 mg q6h or 1 g q12h	D and I	500 mg q6-12h	500 mg q24-48h	500 mg q48-96h	Hemo: Dose for GFR < 10; CAPD: Dose for GFR < 10; CAVH: Dose for GFR 10-50
Vd increases with infection.									

For definitions of the abbreviations used in the tables, see page 14.

Antimicrobial Agents (Continued)

Drug, Toxicity Notes	Percent Excreted Unchanged %	Half-Life (Normal/ ESRD) h	Plasma Protein Binding %	Volume of Distribution L/kg	Dose for Normal Renal Function	Adjustment for Renal Failure Method	GFR, mL/min >50	10-50	<10	Supplement for Dialysis
Penicillins										
Amoxicillin	50-70	0.9-2.3/5-20	15-25	0.26	250-500 mg q8h	I	q8h	q8-12h	q24h	Hemo: Dose after dialysis CAPD: 250 mg q12h CAVH: Not applicable
Ampicillin Sodium, 2.6 mEq/g.	30-90	0.8-1.5/7-20	20	0.17-0.31	250 mg-2 g q6h	I	q6h	q6-12h	q12-24h	Hemo: Dose after dialysis CAPD: 250 mg q12h CAVH: Dose for GFR 10-50
Azlocillin Sodium, 3.0 mEq/g.	50-75	0.8-1.5/5-6	30	0.18-0.27	2-3 g q4h	I	q4-6h	q6-8h	q8h	Hemo: Dose after dialysis CAPD: Dose for GFR < 10 CAVH: Dose for GFR 10-50
Dicloxacillin Sodium, 2.7 mEq/g. May cause hypokalemic metabolic alkalosis.	35-70	0.7/1-2	95	0.16	250-500 mg q6h	D	100%	100%	100%	Hemo: None CAPD: None CAVH: Not applicable
Methicillin	25-80	0.5-1.0/4.0	35-60	0.31	1-2 g q4h	I	q4-6h	q6-8h	q8-12h	Hemo: None CAPD: None CAVH: None
Mezlocillin	65	0.6-1.2/2.6-5.4	20-46	0.18	1.5-4.0 g q4-6h	I	q4-6h	q6-8h	q8h	Hemo: None CAPD: None CAVH: None

Sodium, 1.9 mEq/g. Schedule next dose after dialysis. Reduce dose further for liver and kidney disease.

Drug					Dose		>50	$10-50$	<10	Dialysis
Nafcillin	35	0.5/1.2	85		1-2 g q4-6h	D	100%	100%	100%	Hemo: None CAPD: None CAVH: None
Penicillin G	60-85	0.5/6-20	50	0.3-0.42	0.5-4 million U q6h	D	100%	75%	20-50%	Hemo: Dose after dialysis CAPD: Dose for GFR <10 CAVH: Dose for GFR 10-50
Penicillin VK	60-90	0.6/4.1	50-80	0.5	250 mg q6h	D	100%	100%	100%	Hemo: Dose after dialysis CAPD: Dose for GFR <10 CAVH: Not applicable
Piperacillin	75-90	0.8-1.5/3.3-5.1	30	0.18-0.30	3-4 g q4h	I	q4-6h	q6-8h	q8h	Hemo: Dose after dialysis CAPD: Dose for GFR <10 CAVH: Dose for GFR 10-50
Ticarcillin	85	1.2/11-16	45-60	0.14-0.21	3 g q4h	D and I	1-2 g q4h	1-2 g q8h	1-2 g q12h	Hemo: 3 g after dialysis CAPD: Dose for GFR <10 CAVH: Dose for GFR 10-50

Nafcillin — Coagulopathy.

Penicillin G — Potassium, 1.7 mEq/million units. Seizures. False-positive urine protein reactions. Six million units/d upper limit dose in ESRD.

Piperacillin — Sodium, 1.9 mEq/g.

Ticarcillin — Sodium, 5.2 mEq/g.

Quinolone Antibiotics

Most agents in this group are malabsorbed in the presence of metallic compounds such as magnesium, calcium, aluminum, and iron. Theophylline metabolism is impaired by some of this group. Higher oral doses may be needed to treat CAPD peritonitis.

Drug					Dose		>50	$10-50$	<10	Dialysis
Cinoxacin	55	1.2/12	63	0.25	500 mg q12h	D	100%	50%	Avoid	Hemo: Avoid CAPD: Avoid CAVH: Avoid

For definitions of the abbreviations used in the tables, see page 14.

Antimicrobial Agents (Continued)

Drug, Toxicity Notes	Percent Excreted Unchanged	Half-Life (Normal/ ESRD)	Plasma Protein Binding	Volume of Distribution	Dose for Normal Renal Function	Method	Adjustment for Renal Failure GFR, mL/min >50	10-50	<10	Supplement for Dialysis
	%	h	%	L/kg						
Ciprofloxacin	50-70	3-6/6-9	20-40	2.5	500-750 mg q12h	D	100%	50-75%	50%	Hemo: 250 mg q12h CAPD: 250 mg q8h CAVH: 200 mg iv q12h
Poorly absorbed with antacids, sucralfate, and phosphate binders. Intravenous dose 1/3 of oral dose. Decreases phenytoin levels.										
Fleroxacin	70	13/21-28	20	1.1-2.4	400 mg q12h	D	100%	50-75%	50%	Hemo: 400 mg after dialysis CAPD: 400 mg/d CAVH: Not applicable
Lomefloxacin	76	8/44	15	1.8-3.1	400 mg/d	D	100%	50-75%	50%	Hemo: Dose for GFR < 10 CAPD: Dose for GFR < 10 CAVH: Not applicable
Nalidixic acid	High	6/21	90	0.25-0.35	1.0 g q6h	D	100%	Avoid	Avoid	Hemo: Avoid CAPD: Avoid CAVH: Not applicable
Norfloxacin	30	3.5-6.5/8	14	< 0.5	400 mg q12h	I	q12h	q12-24h	Avoid	Hemo: Not applicable CAPD: Not applicable CAVH: Not applicable
Ofloxacin	68-80	5-8/28-37	25	1.5-2.5	400 mg/d	D	100%	50%	25-50%	Hemo: 100 mg bid CAPD: Dose for GFR < 10 CAVH: 300 mg/d

						GFR >50	GFR 10-50	GFR <10	
Pefloxacin	11	10/15	25-43	2	400 mg/d	D	100%	100%	100%	Hemo: None CAPD: None CAVH: None

Excellent bidirectional transperitoneal movement.

Tetracycline Antibiotics

Potentiate acidosis. Increase BUN, phosphorus. Antianabolic.

Doxycycline	33-45	15-24/18-25	80-93	0.75	100 mg/d	D	100%	100%	100%	Hemo: None CAPD: None CAVH: None

Group drug of choice for decreased renal function. Not antianabolic.

Minocycline	6-10	12-16/12-18	70	1.0-1.5	100 mg q12h	D	100%	100%	100%	Hemo: None CAPD: None CAVH: None

Tetracycline	48-60	6-10/57-108	55-90	> 0.7	250-500 mg qid	I	q8-12h	q12-24h	q24h	Hemo: None CAPD: None CAVH: None

Avoid in ESRD.

Antifungal Antibiotics

Amphotericin	5	24/Unchanged	90	4	20-40 mg/d	I	q24h	q24h	q24-36h	Hemo: None CAPD: Dose for GFR < 10 CAVH: Dose for GFR 10-50

Nephrotoxic. Renal tubular acidosis, potassium wasting. Nephrogenic diabetes insipidus. Ineffective for UTI in ESRD. Toxicity lessened by saline loading and worsened by concomitant cyclosporin A, aminoglycosides, or pentamidine.

For definitions of the abbreviations used in the tables, see page 14.

31

Antimicrobial Agents (Continued)

Drug, Toxicity Notes	Percent Excreted Unchanged	Half-Life (Normal/ESRD)	Plasma Protein Binding	Volume of Distribution	Dose for Normal Renal Function	Adjustment for Renal Failure				Supplement for Dialysis
						Method	GFR, mL/min			
							>50	10-50	<10	
	%	h	%	L/kg						
Fluconazole	70	22/Unknown	12	0.7	200-400 mg/d	D	100%	100%	100%	Hemo: 200 mg after dialysis CAPD: Dose for GFR < 10 CAVH: Dose for GFR 10-50
Flucytosine	90	3-6/75-200	< 10	0.6	37.5 mg/kg q6h	I	q12h	q16h	q24h	Hemo: Dose after dialysis CAPD: 0.5-1.0 g/d CAVH: Dose for GFR 10-50
Griseofulvin Hepatic dysfunction. Therapeutic goal level of 75 mg/L. Marrow suppression more common in azotemic patients.	1	14/20	Unknown	1.6	125-250 mg q6h	D	100%	100%	100%	Hemo: None CAPD: None CAVH: None
Itraconazole	35	21/25	99	10	100-200 mg q12h	D	100%	100%	50-100%	Hemo: 100 mg q12-24h CAPD: 100 mg q12-24h CAVH: 100 mg q12-24h
Ketoconazole	13	1.5-3.3/3.3	99	1.9-3.6	200 mg/d	D	100%	100%	100%	Hemo: None CAPD: None CAVH: None
Miconazole	1	20-24/Unchanged	90	Large	200-1200 mg q8h	D	100%	100%	100%	Hemo: None CAPD: None CAVH: None

Antiparasitic Antibiotics

Drug										Supplement
Chloroquine	40	2-4/5-50 d	50-65	Large	1.5 g over 3 d	D	100%	100%	50%	Hemo: None CAPD: None CAVH: None

Excretion increased in alkaline urine.

Pentamidine	20	29/118	69	55-462	4 mg/kg · d	I	q24h	q24-36h	q48h	Hemo: None CAPD: None CAVH: None

Extensive tissue uptake. Nephrotoxic. Hyperkalemia.

Pyrimethamine	16-30	80/Unchanged	27	2.9	50-75 mg/d	D	100%	100%	100%	Hemo: None CAPD: None CAVH: None

Metabolites excreted for weeks because of tissue deposition. Doses are for treatment of toxoplasmosis. Antimalarial doses much lower.

Quinine	5-20	5-16/Unchanged	70	0.7-3.7	650 mg q8h	I	q8h	q8-12h	q24h	Hemo: Dose after dialysis CAPD: Dose for GFR < 10 CAVH: Dose for GFR 10-50

Marked tissue accumulation.

Antituberculous Antibiotics

Capreomycin	50	2	Unknown	Unknown	1 g/d	I	q24h	q24h	q48h	Hemo: None CAPD: None CAVH: None

Nephrotoxic. Potentiates neuromuscular blockade.

For definitions of the abbreviations used in the tables, see page 14.

Antimicrobial Agents (Continued)

Drug, Toxicity Notes	Percent Excreted Unchanged	Half-Life (Normal/ESRD)	Plasma Protein Binding	Volume of Distribution	Dose for Normal Renal Function	Adjustment for Renal Failure Method	GFR, mL/min >50	10-50	<10	Supplement for Dialysis
	%	h	%	L/kg						
Cycloserine CNS toxicity.	65	0.5	Unknown	0.11-0.26	250 mg q12h	I	q12h	q12-24h	q24h	Hemo: None CAPD: None CAVH: None
Ethambutol Decreases visual acuity. Peripheral neuritis.	75-90	4/7-15	10-30	1.6-3.2	15 mg/kg · d	I	q24h	q24-36h	q48h	Hemo: Dose after dialysis CAPD: Dose for GFR < 10 CAVH: Dose for GFR 10-50
Ethionamide	1	2.1	30	Unknown	250-500 mg q12h	D	100%	100%	50%	Hemo: None CAPD: None CAVH: None
Isoniazide Dosing is for slow acetylators.	5-30	0.7-4/8-17	4-30	0.75	5 mg/kg · d	D	100%	100%	50%	Hemo: Dose after dialysis CAPD: Dose for GFR < 10 CAVH: Dose for GFR < 10
PAS Significant sodium load.	80	1	15-50	0.11-0.24	50 mg/kg q8h	D	100%	50-75%	50%	Hemo: Dose after dialysis CAPD: Dose for GFR < 10 CAVH: Dose for GFR < 10
Pyrazinimide Impairs urate excretion. Can precipitate gout.	1-3	9/26	5	0.75-1.3	25 kg/d	D	100%	Avoid	Avoid	Hemo: Avoid CAPD: Avoid CAVH: Avoid

				Dose	D	100%	50-100%	50%	Supplement
Rifampin	15-30	1.5-5/1.8-11	60-90	0.9	600 mg/d					Hemo: None CAPD: Dose for GFR < 10 CAVH: Dose for GFR < 10

Acute interstitial nephritis. Potassium wasting. Renal tubular defects. Biologically active metabolite.

Antiviral Agents

					Dose	D	100%	50-100%	50%	Supplement
Acyclovir	40-70	2.1-3.8/20	15-30	0.7	5 mg/kg q8h	D and I	5 mg/kg q8h	5 mg/kg q12-24h	2.5 mg/kg q24h	Hemo: Dose after dialysis CAPD: Dose for GFR < 10 CAVH: 3.5 mg/kg · d

Neurotoxicity in ESRD. Intravenous preparation can cause renal failure if injected rapidly.

					Dose	D	100%	50-100%	50%	Supplement
Amantadine	90	12/500	60	4-5	100 mg q12h	I	q24-48h	q48-72h	q7d	Hemo: None CAPD: None CAVH: None
Didanosine	40	1.6/?	Unknown	1.0	100-300 mg q12h	I	q12h	q24h	q48h	Hemo: Dose after dialysis CAPD: Dose for GFR < 10 CAVH: Dose for GFR < 10

ESRD dosing guidelines are estimates.

					Dose	D	100%	50-100%	50%	Supplement
Foscarnet	85	3/Prolonged	17	0.3-0.6	60 mg/kg q8h induction doses only	D	28 mg/kg q8h	15 mg/kg q8h	6 mg/kg q8h	Hemo: Dose after dialysis CAPD: Dose for GFR < 10 CAVH: Dose for GFR 10-50

Nephrotoxic; seizures, hypokalemia, hypocalcemia, hypomagnesemia.

					Dose	D	100%	50-100%	50%	Supplement
Ganciclovir	90-100	3.6/30	Unknown	0.47	5 mg/kg q12h	I	q12h	q24-48h	q48-96h	Hemo: Dose after dialysis CAPD: Dose for GFR < 10 CAVH: 2.5 mg/kg · d

Marrow toxicity.

For definitions of the abbreviations used in the tables, see page 14.

Antimicrobial Agents (Continued)

Drug, Toxicity Notes	Percent Excreted Unchanged	Half-Life (Normal/ESRD)	Plasma Protein Binding	Volume of Distribution	Dose for Normal Renal Function	Adjustment for Renal Failure				Supplement for Dialysis
						Method	GFR, *mL/min*			
							>50	10-50	<10	
	%	h	%	L/kg						
Ribavirin	10-40	30-60/Unknown	0	9-15	200 mg q8h	D	100%	100%	50%	Hemo: Dose after dialysis CAPD: Dose for GFR < 10 CAVH: Dose for GFR < 10
Half-life data from multiple doses. Loading dose required. Oral absorption 40%.										
Vidarabine	50	1.5/Unknown	25	0.7	15 mg/kg infusion q24h	D	100%	100%	75%	Hemo: Infuse after dialysis CAPD: Dose for GFR < 10 CAVH: Dose for GFR 10-50
Active metabolite excreted by the kidney.										
Zidovudine (AZT)	8-25	1.1-1.4/1.4-3	10-30	1.4-3	200 mg q8h	D and I	200 mg q8h	200 mg q8h	100 mg q12h	Hemo: 100 mg after dialysis CAPD: Dose for GFR < 10 CAVH: 100 mg q8h
Enormous interpatient variation. Marrow suppression.										

Antihypertensive and Cardiovascular Agents

Hypertension and coronary heart disease occur frequently in patients with impaired renal function. Antihypertensive and cardiovascular agents are the most commonly prescribed drugs in patients with renal disease. Narrow therapeutic range and individual variability in drug response complicate the use of these drugs. As shown in the table, some of these drugs or their metabolites accumulate in patients with renal insufficiency, and abnormalities of drug binding to plasma proteins may make more free drug available at receptor sites, enhancing both drug efficacy and toxicity.

The relation between renal drug elimination and the cardiovascular system is well established. Drugs may alter their own elimination rate or their effect on the kidneys by improving cardiac output and effective renal blood flow. For example, patients with decompensated congestive heart failure may be resistant to diuretics. If natriuresis can be initiated, the subsequent improvement in cardiovascular function can increase response to the diuretic. Thus, the effect of cardiovascular drugs may also vary among patients as cardiac function changes.

The use of antiarrhythmic agents requires that special care be taken. Because toxicity may appear as the same arrhythmia the drug is intended to correct, recognition of toxicity may be delayed. Inappropriate increases in antiarrhythmic dose may be fatal. Monitoring other electrocardiographic evidence of toxicity, such as a prolonged Q-T interval or widening of the QRS complex, may be essential to proper diagnosis.

Procainamide causes particular problems in patients with renal dysfunction. The elimination of the drug is slowed by renal failure; the excretion of its primary metabolite, N-acetyl procainamide, depends on kidney function; and the parent drug and metabolite appear to have different antiarrhythmic spectra and elimination rates. Avoiding procainamide in patients with renal impairment would seem prudent, but this approach is often not practical. Careful monitoring is essential, and measurement of drug and metabolite levels may be helpful.

Many antihypertensive agents are excreted by the kidney. Because of the wide variability of drug response among patients, the response of blood pressure to dose must be monitored for each patient. Steady-state drug levels are usually not achieved until after the drug has been given for at least three or four half-lives. The data in the table may be useful in predicting the best time for changing the dose during the titration process.

Diuretics remain an essential part of most antihypertensive therapy and can be grouped into two categories on the basis of their clinical use. The potassium-sparing drugs, amiloride, spirono-lactone, and triamterene, may produce hyperkalemia in patients with creatinine clearance rates below 30 mL/min and should be avoided in these patients. The remaining diuretics are organic acids and need to reach the tubular lumen to be active. In patients with impaired renal function, endogenous organic acids accumu-late and compete with diuretics for secretion into the tubular lumen. Consequently, as renal function decreases, larger doses of diuretics are required. As the glomerular filtration rate falls, the thiazides become ineffective. However, large doses of the loop diuretics, furosemide, bumetanide, or ethacrynic acid, may still produce diuresis. In patients with renal insufficiency, diuretic-induced dehydration may result in a further loss of renal function. Unless patients require diuresis for substantial peripheral edema or congestive heart failure, hypertension in patients with decreased renal function should be managed so as to avoid unnecessary volume contraction.

Each of the antihypertensive drugs listed in the table can be toxic. The adverse effects are generally related to pharmacologic effect and can be avoided by careful dose titration. The develop-ment of newer, effective antihypertensive agents makes more individualized pharmacotherapy possible. Choosing an antihyper-tensive agent should include understanding the altered homeo-static mechanisms in patients with impaired renal function.

When blood pressure is appropriately lowered in hypertensive patients with renal insufficiency, a transient decrease in renal function may occur. As hypertensive microvascular changes im-prove, renal function should again increase. In some cases dialysis may be needed temporarily. If renal function decreases with antihypertensive therapy and does not improve, drug-related nephrotoxicity or another potentially reversible cause should be considered.

The choice of cardiac glycosides in patients with renal insufficiency is controversial. Digoxin is excreted by the kidneys, and dosages must be reduced substantially for patients with modest decreases in renal function. Because digitoxin is excreted primarily by the liver, dosage reduction is required only in patients with severe renal impairment. However, digitoxin's long half-life makes toxicity with this drug potentially more serious. Both drugs have been reported to have a smaller volume of distribution in patients with renal insufficiency, making calculation of the appropriate loading dose more difficult. When digitalization can be done gradually, a small loading dose followed by reduced maintenance doses is preferred.

Antihypertensive and Cardiovascular Agents

Drug, Toxicity Notes	Percent Excreted Unchanged	Half-Life (Normal/ ESRD)	Plasma Protein Binding	Volume of Distribution	Dose for Normal Renal Function	Adjustment for Renal Failure				Supplement for Dialysis
						Method	GFR, mL/min			
							>50	10-50	<10	
	%	h	%	L/kg						

Antihypertensive Drugs

Blood pressure is the best guide to dose and interval.

Adrenergic and Serotoninergic Modulators

| Clonidine | 45 | 6-23/39-42 | 20-40 | 3-6 | 0.1-0.6 mg bid | D | 100% | 100% | 100% | Hemo: None
CAPD: None
CAVH: Unknown |

Rebound hypertension if drug is abruptly withdrawn. Tricyclic antidepressants decrease efficacy. Potentiates CNS depressant effects of alcohol, sedatives.

| Doxazosin | < 5 | 9.5-12.5/13 | 98 | 1-1.7 | 1-16 mg/d | D | 100% | 100% | 100% | Hemo: None
CAPD: None
CAVH: Unknown |

Renal patients may be sensitive to small doses, similar to prazosin.

| Guanabenz | < 5 | 12-14/Unknown | 90 | 10-12 | 8-16 mg bid | D | 100% | 100% | 100% | Hemo: Unknown
CAPD: Unknown
CAVH: Unknown |

Similar to clonidine.

| Guanadrel | 30-40 | 4-10/19 | 20 | 11.5 | 10-50 mg bid | I | q12h | q12-24h | q24-48h | Hemo: Unknown
CAPD: Unknown
CAVH: Unknown |

Similar to guanethidine, but less diarrhea.

Drug				Dose	D/I				Supplement
Guanethidine	25-50	120-140/Unknown	<5	Unknown	10-100 mg/d	I	q24h	q24h	q24-36h	Hemo: Unknown CAPD: Unknown CAVH: Unknown
Tricyclic antidepressants decrease efficacy. Cause orthostatic hypotension, diarrhea.										
Guanfacine	24-37	12-23/15-25	65	4-6.5	1-2 mg/d	D	100%	100%	100%	Hemo: None CAPD: None CAVH: Unknown
Similar to clonidine, but milder.										
Ketanserin	<2	14-19/25-35	95	3-6	40 mg bid	D	100%	100%	100%	Hemo: None CAPD: None CAVH: Unknown
Serotonin receptor antagonist; protein binding decreased in uremia.										
Methyldopa	25-40	1.5-6/6-16	<15	0.5	250-500 mg tid	I	q8h	q8-12h	q12-24h	Hemo: 250 mg CAPD: None CAVH: Unknown
Orthostatic hypotension. Retroperitoneal fibrosis. Interferes with serum creatinine measurement. Active metabolites with long half-life.										
Prazosin	<5	2-3/2-3	97	1.2-1.5	1-15 mg bid	D	100%	100%	100%	Hemo: None CAPD: None CAVH: Unknown
May produce profound first-dose hypotension. Renal patients should be titrated starting from low doses.										
Reserpine	<1	46-168/87-323	96	Unknown	0.05-0.25 mg/d	D	100%	100%	Avoid	Hemo: None CAPD: None CAVH: Unknown
Excessive sedation. Gastrointestinal bleeding.										
Terazosin	20-30	9-12/8-12	90-94	0.5-0.9	1-20 mg/d	D	100%	100%	100%	Hemo: None CAPD: Unknown CAVH: Unknown
Similar to prazosin.										

For definitions of the abbreviations used in the tables, see page 14.

Antihypertensive and Cardiovascular Agents (Continued)

Drug, Toxicity Notes	Percent Excreted Unchanged %	Half-Life (Normal/ ESRD) h	Plasma Protein Binding %	Volume of Distribution L/kg	Dose for Normal Renal Function	Adjustment for Renal Failure Method	Adjustment for Renal Failure GFR, mL/min >50	Adjustment for Renal Failure GFR, mL/min 10-50	Adjustment for Renal Failure GFR, mL/min <10	Supplement for Dialysis

Angiotensin-Converting Enzyme Inhibitors

Hypotensive effects magnified by natriuretic agents or sodium depletion. Can cause hyperkalemia, metabolic acidosis. Acute renal dysfunction with bilateral or transplant renal artery stenosis, low renal perfusion pressure. Dry cough in 5-10%.

Drug, Toxicity Notes	Percent Excreted Unchanged %	Half-Life (Normal/ ESRD) h	Plasma Protein Binding %	Volume of Distribution L/kg	Dose for Normal Renal Function	Method	>50	10-50	<10	Supplement for Dialysis
Benazepril	20	22/30	95	1.5	10 mg/d	D	100%	75-100%	50%	Hemo: 25-30% CAPD: None CAVH: Unknown
Benazeprilat, the active moeity formed in liver.										
Captopril	30-40	1.9/21-32	25-30	0.7-3	25 mg q8h	D and I	100% q8-12h	75% q12-18h	50% q24h	Hemo: 25-35% CAPD: None CAVH: Unknown
Rare proteinuria, nephrotic syndrome, dysgeusia, granulocytopenia. Increases serum digoxin levels.										
Enalapril	43	11-24/34-60	50-60	Unknown	5-10 mg q12h	D	100%	75-100%	50%	Hemo: 20-25% CAPD: None CAVH: Unknown
Enalaprilat, the active moeity formed in liver.										
Fosinopril	< 1	11.5-12/12-20	95	1.5	10 mg/d	D	100%	100%	75%	Hemo: None CAPD: None CAVH Unknown
Fosinoprilat, the active moeity formed in liver. Drug less likely than other angiotensin-converting enzyme inhibitors to accumulate in renal failure.										

Drug					Dose	Method				Supplement
Lisinopril	80-90	12.6/40-50	0-10	1.3-1.5	5-10 mg/d	D	100%	50-75%	25-50%	Hemo: 20% CAPD: None CAVH: Unknown
Quinapril	30	1-2/6-15	97	1.5	10-20 mg/d	D	100%	75-100%	50%	Hemo: 25% CAPD: None CAVH: Unknown
Ramipril	10-21	5-8/15	55-70	Unknown	10-20 mg/d	D	100%	50-75%	25-50%	Hemo: 20% CAPD: None CAVH: Unknown

Lisinopril: Lysine analog of the active enalapril metabolite.

Quinapril: Quinalaprilat, the active moeity formed in the liver.

Ramipril: Ramiprilat, the active moeity formed in liver.

Beta Blockers

Drug					Dose	Method				Supplement
Acebutolol	55	7-9/7	20	1.2	400-600 mg/d or bid	D	100%	50%	30-50%	Hemo: None CAPD: None CAVH: Unknown
Atenolol	>90%	6.7/15-35	3	1.1	50-100 mg/d	D and I	100% q24h	50% q48h	30-50% q96h	Hemo: 25-50 mg CAPD: None CAVH: Unknown
Betaxolol	80-90	15-20/30-35	45-60	5-10	20 mg/d	D	100%	100%	50%	Hemo: None CAPD: None CAVH: Unknown
Bopindolol	<10	4-10/Unchanged	Unknown	2-3	1-4 mg/d	D	100%	100%	100%	Hemo: None CAPD: None CAVH: Unknown

Acebutolol: Hyperkalemia in ESRD.

Atenolol: Active metabolites with long half-life.

Betaxolol: Accumulates in ESRD.

Bopindolol: Predrug hydrolysed rapidly to active metabolite.

For definitions of the abbreviations used in the tables, see page 14.

Antihypertensive and Cardiovascular Agents (Continued)

Drug, Toxicity Notes	Percent Excreted Unchanged	Half-Life (Normal/ ESRD)	Plasma Protein Binding	Volume of Distribution	Dose for Normal Renal Function	Method	Adjustment for Renal Failure GFR, mL/min >50	10-50	<10	Supplement for Dialysis
	%	h	%	L/kg						
Carteolol	> 50	7/33	20-30	4	0.5-10 mg/d	D	100%	50%	25%	Hemo: Unknown CAPD: None CAVH: Unknown
Celiprolol	10	4-5/5	Unknown	Unknown	200 mg/d	D	100%	100%	75%	Hemo: Unknown CAPD: None CAVH: Unknown
Dilevalol	< 5	8-12/19-30	75	25	400-600 mg bid	D	100%	100%	100%	Hemo: None CAPD: None CAVH: Unknown
Esmolol	< 10	7-15 min/Unchanged	55	3	50-150 μg/kg · min by infusion	D	100%	100%	100%	Hemo: None CAPD: None CAVH: Unknown
Inactive metabolite accumulates.										
Labetolol	< 5	3-9/Unchanged	50	5.6	200-600 mg bid	D	100%	100%	100%	Hemo: None CAPD: None CAVH: Unknown
Metoprolol	5	3.5/2.5-4.5	8	5.5	50-100 mg bid	D	100%	100%	100%	Hemo: 50 mg CAPD: None CAVH: Unknown

Nadolol	90	19/45	28	1.9	80-120 mg/d	D	100%	50%	25%	Hemo: 40 mg CAPD: None CAVH: Unknown
Penbutolol	<10	22/24	>95	Unknown	10-40 mg/d	D	100%	100%	100%	Hemo: None CAPD: None CAVH: Unknown
Pindolol	40	2.5-4/3-4	50	1.2	10-40 mg bid	D	100%	100%	100%	Hemo: None CAPD: None CAVH: Unknown
Propranolol	<5	2-6/1-6	93	2.8	80-160 mg bid	D	100%	100%	100%	Hemo: None CAPD: None CAVH: Unknown
	Bioavailability may increase. Metabolites may cause increased bilirubin by assay interference. Hypoglycemia reported in ESRD.									
Sotalol	60	7.5-15/56	<1	1.3	160 mg/d	D	100%	30%	15-30%	Hemo: 80 mg CAPD: None CAVH: Unknown
Timolol	15	2.7/4	60	1.7	10-20 mg bid	D	100%	100%	100%	Hemo: None CAPD: None CAVH: Unknown
Vasodilators										
Diazoxide	50	17-31/30-60	>90	0.2-0.3	150-300 mg bolus	D	100%	100%	100%	Hemo: None CAPD: None CAVH: Not applicable
	Sodium and water retention.									

For definitions of the abbreviations used in the tables, see page 14.

Antihypertensive and Cardiovascular Agents (Continued)

Drug, Toxicity Notes	Percent Excreted Unchanged	Half-Life (Normal/ESRD)	Plasma Protein Binding	Volume of Distribution	Dose for Normal Renal Function	Adjustment for Renal Failure				Supplement for Dialysis
						Method	GFR, mL/min			
							>50	10-50	<10	
	%	h	%	L/kg						
Hydralazine	25	2-4.5/7-16	87	0.5-0.9	25-50 mg tid	I	q8h	q8h	q8-16h	Hemo: None CAPD: None CAVH: Unknown
Drug-induced lupus.										
Minoxidil	15-20	2.8-4.2/Unchanged	0	2-3	5-30 mg bid	D	100%	100%	100%	Hemo: None CAPD: None CAVH: Unknown
Fluid retention, pericardial effusion.										
Nitroprusside	<10	<10 min/<10 min	0	0.2	0.25-8 µg/kg · min by infusion	D	100%	100%	100%	Hemo: None CAPD: None CAVH: Unknown
Toxic metabolite, thiocyanate, accumulates causing seizures, coma. Thiocyanate is hemodialyzable. Measure thiocyanate levels. Sodium thiosulfate effective in treatment.										

Antiarrhythmic Agents

Blood levels most often the best guide to therapy. Half-life may be prolonged in heart failure or with reduced hepatic blood flow.

Drug					Dose	Method	>50	10-50	<10	Supplement
Adenosine	<5	<10 sec/Unchanged	0	?	3-6 mg iv bolus	D	100%	100%	100%	Hemo: None / CAPD: None / CAVH: No data
Amiodarone	<5	14-120 d/Unchanged	96	70-140	800-2000 mg load 200-600 mg/d	D	100%	100%	100%	Hemo: None / CAPD: None / CAVH: No data

Hepatotoxicity. Thyroid dysfunction. Peripheral neuropathy. Pulmonary fibrosis. Active metabolite. Increased plasma digoxin. Increases cyclosporine levels.

Drug					Dose	Method	>50	10-50	<10	Supplement
Bretylium	75	6-13.6/16-32	6	8.2	5-30 mg/kg load 5-10 mg iv q6h	D	100%	25-50%	25%	Hemo: None / CAPD: None / CAVH: No data

Hypotension. Active metabolites.

Drug					Dose	Method	>50	10-50	<10	Supplement
Cibenzoline	50-60	7/22	50	4-5	130-160 mg q12h	D and I	100% q12h	100% q24h	66% q24h	Hemo: None / CAPD: None / CAVH: No data
Disopyramide	35-65	5-8/10-18	54-81	0.8-2.6	100-200 mg q6h	I	q8h	q12-24h	q24-40h	Hemo: None / CAPD: None / CAVH: No data

Urinary retention. Protein binding concentration dependent. Volume of distribution decreased in ESRD.

For definitions of the abbreviations used in the tables, see page 14.

Antihypertensive and Cardiovascular Agents (Continued)

Drug, Toxicity Notes	Percent Excreted Unchanged	Half-Life (Normal/ ESRD)	Plasma Protein Binding	Volume of Distribution	Dose for Normal Renal Function	Adjustment for Renal Failure Method	GFR, mL/min >50	GFR, mL/min 10-50	GFR, mL/min <10	Supplement for Dialysis
	%	h	%	L/kg						
Encainide	70-85	3-9/1.5-9	75-81	2-2.7	25 mg q8h to 50 mg q6h	D	100%	75%	50%	Hemo: No data CAPD: No data CAVH: No data
Encephalopathy. Slow demethylators with long half-life. Active metabolite.										
Flecainide	25	12-19.5/19-26	52	8.4-9.5	100 mg q12h to 350-400 mg prn	D	100%	100%	50-75%	Hemo: None CAPD: None CAVH: No data
Excretion enhanced in acid urine.										
Lidocaine	10	2-2.2/1.3-3	60-66	1.3-2.2	50 mg over 2 min, repeat q5min × 3, then 1-4 mg/min	D	100%	100%	100%	Hemo: None CAPD: None CAVH: No data
Lorcainide	< 2	9/Unknown	80-85	10	100 mg bid	D	100%	100%	100%	Hemo: No data CAPD: No data CAVH: No data
Active metabolite.										
Mexiletine	10	8-13/16	70-75	5.5-6.6	100-300 mg q6-12h	D	100%	100%	50-75%	Hemo: None CAPD: None CAVH: None
Increased renal excretion in acid urine.										
Moricizine	< 1	2/3	95	> 5	200-300 q8h	D	100%	100%	100%	Hemo: None CAPD: None CAVH: No data

						GFR >50	GFR 10-50	GFR <10	
N-Acetyl-procainamide	80	6-8/42-70	10-20	1.5-1.7	500 mg q6-8h	D and I	100% q6-8h	50% q8-12h	25% q12-18h	Hemo: None CAPD: None CAVH: Replace by blood level

Hemofiltration useful in poisoning.

Procainamide	50-60	2.5-4.9/5.3-5.9	15	2.2	350-400 mg q3-4h	I	q4h	q6-12h	q8-24h	Hemo: 200 mg CAPD: None CAVH: Replace by blood level

Half-life acetylator phenotype dependent. Active metabolite is *N*-acetyl-procainamide. Lupus-like syndrome. Hemofiltration useful in poisoning.

Propafenone	<1	5/Unknown	>95	3	150-300 mg q8h	D	100%	100%	100%	Hemo: None CAPD: None CAVH: No data

Half-life acetylator phenotype dependent. Active metabolite.

Quinidine	20	6/4-14	70-95	2-3.5	200-400 mg q4-6h	D	100%	100%	75%	Hemo: 100-200 mg CAPD: None CAVH: No data

Active metabolite. Increased plasma levels of digoxin and digitoxin. Excretion enhanced in acid urine. Hemodialysis useful in poisoning.

Tocainide	40	14/22-27	10-20	3.2	200-400 mg q4-6h	D	100%	100%	50%	Hemo: 200 mg CAPD: None CAVH: No data

Excretion decreased in alkaline urine.

Calcium Channel Blockers

Headache, flushing, dizziness. May increase digoxin and cyclosporine levels.

Amlodipine	<10	35-50/50	>95	21	5 mg/d	D	100%	100%	100%	Hemo: None CAPD: None CAVH: No data

For definitions of the abbreviations used in the tables, see page 14.

Antihypertensive and Cardiovascular Agents (Continued)

Drug, Toxicity Notes	Percent Excreted Unchanged	Half-Life (Normal/ESRD)	Plasma Protein Binding	Volume of Distribution	Dose for Normal Renal Function	Adjustment for Renal Failure				Supplement for Dialysis
						Method	GFR, mL/min			
							>50	10-50	<10	
	%	h	%	L/kg						
Diltiazem	< 10	2-8/3.5	98	3-5	90 mg q8h	D	100%	100%	100%	Hemo: None CAPD: None CAVH: No data
Active metabolites. Acute renal dysfunction reported.										
Felodipine	< 1	10-14/21-24	99	9-10	10 mg/d	D	100%	100%	100%	Hemo: None CAPD: None CAVH: No data
Isradipine	< 5	1.9-4.8/10-11	97	3-4	5-10 mg/d	D	100%	100%	100%	Hemo: None CAPD: None CAVH: No data
Nicardipine	< 1	5/5-7	98-99	0.8	20-30 mg tid	D	100%	100%	100%	Hemo: None CAPD: None CAVH: No data
Uremia inhibits hepatic metabolism.										
Nifedipine	< 10	4-5.5/5-7	97	1.4	10-20 mg q6-8h	D	100%	100%	100%	Hemo: None CAPD: None CAVH: No data
Acute renal dysfunction reported. Protein binding decreased in ESRD.										
Nimodipine	< 10	1-2.8/22	98	0.9-2.3	30 mg q8h	D	100%	100%	100%	Hemo: None CAPD: None CAVH: No data
May lower blood pressure.										

Drug									
Nisoldipine	<10	6.6-7.9/6.8-9.7	99	2.3-7.1	10 mg bid	D	100%	100%	100%	Hemo: None CAPD: None CAVH: No data
Nitrendipine	<1	4.6/3.3-5.8	99	6.6	20 mg bid	D	100%	100%	100%	Hemo: None CAPD: None CAVH: No data
Verapamil	<10	3-7/2.4-4	83-93	3-6	80 mg q8h	D	100%	100%	100%	Hemo: None CAPD: None CAVH: No data

Acute renal dysfunction reported. Active metabolites accumulate particularly with sustained release forms.

Cardiac Glycosides

Add to uremic gastrointestinal symptoms. Toxicity enhanced by hypokalemia and hypomagnesemia during dialysis.

Digitoxin	20-25	144-200/210	94	0.6	0.1-0.2 mg/d	D	100%	100%	50-75%	Hemo: None CAPD: None CAVH: No data

8-10% converted to digoxin. More converted to digoxin in ESRD. Volume of distribution decreased by uremia.

Digoxin	76-85	36-44/80-120	20-30	5-8	1-1.5 mg load 0.25-0.5 mg/d	D and I	100% q24h	25-75% q36h	10-25% q48h	Hemo: None CAPD: None CAVH: 0.5 mg q12h

Decrease loading dose by 50% in ESRD. Radioimmunoassay may overestimate serum levels in uremia. Clearance decreased by amiodarone, spironolactone, quinidine, verapamil. Hypokalemia, hypomagnesemia enhance toxicity. Volume of distribution and total body clearance decreased in ESRD. Serum level 12 hours after dose is best guide in ESRD. Digoxin immune antibodies can treat severe toxicity in ESRD.

For definitions of the abbreviations used in the tables, see page 14.

Antihypertensive and Cardiovascular Agents (Continued)

Drug, Toxicity Notes	Percent Excreted Unchanged %	Half-Life (Normal/ ESRD) h	Plasma Protein Binding %	Volume of Distribution L/kg	Dose for Normal Renal Function	Adjustment for Renal Failure Method	Adjustment for Renal Failure GFR, mL/min >50	Adjustment for Renal Failure GFR, mL/min 10-50	Adjustment for Renal Failure GFR, mL/min <10	Supplement for Dialysis
Ouabain	40-50	21/60-70	40	Unknown	0.25 mg load 0.1 mg q12h	I	q12-24h	q24-36h	q36-48h	Hemo: None CAPD: None CAVH: No data

Diuretics

Natriuretic drugs may cause extracellular fluid volume depletion.

Drug, Toxicity Notes	Percent Excreted Unchanged %	Half-Life (Normal/ ESRD) h	Plasma Protein Binding %	Volume of Distribution L/kg	Dose for Normal Renal Function	Adjustment for Renal Failure Method	Adjustment for Renal Failure GFR, mL/min >50	Adjustment for Renal Failure GFR, mL/min 10-50	Adjustment for Renal Failure GFR, mL/min <10	Supplement for Dialysis
Acetazolamide	100	1.7-5.8/Unknown	70-90	0.2	250 mg q6-12h	I	q6h	q12h	Avoid	Hemo: No data CAPD: No data CAVH: None

May potentiate acidosis. Ineffective in ESRD.

Drug, Toxicity Notes	Percent Excreted Unchanged %	Half-Life (Normal/ ESRD) h	Plasma Protein Binding %	Volume of Distribution L/kg	Dose for Normal Renal Function	Adjustment for Renal Failure Method	Adjustment for Renal Failure GFR, mL/min >50	Adjustment for Renal Failure GFR, mL/min 10-50	Adjustment for Renal Failure GFR, mL/min <10	Supplement for Dialysis
Amiloride	50	6-8/10-144	30-40	5-5.2	5 mg/d	D	100%	50%	Avoid	Hemo: Not applicable CAPD: Not applicable CAVH: Not applicable

Hyperkalemia with GFR < 30 mL/min, especially in diabetics. Hyperchloremic metabolic acidosis.

Drug, Toxicity Notes	Percent Excreted Unchanged %	Half-Life (Normal/ ESRD) h	Plasma Protein Binding %	Volume of Distribution L/kg	Dose for Normal Renal Function	Adjustment for Renal Failure Method	Adjustment for Renal Failure GFR, mL/min >50	Adjustment for Renal Failure GFR, mL/min 10-50	Adjustment for Renal Failure GFR, mL/min <10	Supplement for Dialysis
Bumetanide	33	1.2-1.5/1.5	96	0.2-0.5	1-2 mg q8-12h	D	100%	100%	100%	Hemo: None CAPD: None CAVH: Not applicable

Ototoxicity in combination with aminoglycosides. High doses effective in ESRD. Muscle pain, gynecomastia.

Drug	% Excreted Unchanged	Half-Life Normal/ESRD	Plasma Protein Binding (%)	Volume of Distribution	Dose	Method	GFR >50	GFR 10–50	GFR <10	Dialysis
Chlorthalidone	50	44-80/Unknown	76-90	3.9	25 mg/d	I	q24h	q24h	Avoid	Hemo: Not applicable CAPD: Not applicable CAVH: Not applicable
Ethacrynic acid	20	2-4/Unknown	90	0.1	50-100 mg tid	I	q8-12h	q8-12h	Avoid	Hemo: None CAPD: None CAVH: Not applicable
Furosemide	67	0.5-1.1/2-4	95	0.07-0.2	40-80 mg bid	D	100%	100%	100%	Hemo: None CAPD: None CAVH: Not applicable
Indapamide	<5	14-18/Unchanged	76-79	0.3-1.3	2.5 mg/d	D	100%	100%	Avoid	Hemo: None CAPD: None CAVH: Not applicable
Metolazone	70	4-20/Unknown	95	1.6	5-10 mg/d	D	100%	100%	100%	Hemo: None CAPD: None CAVH: Not applicable
Piretanide	40-60	1.4/1.6-3.4	94	0.3	6-12 mg/d	D	100%	100%	100%	Hemo: None CAPD: None CAVH: Not applicable
Spironolactone	20-30	10-35/Unchanged	98	Unknown	25 mg tid-qid	I	q6-12h	q12-24h	Avoid	Hemo: Not applicable CAPD: Not applicable CAVH: Not applicable
Thiazides	>95	6-8/12-20	40	3	25-50 mg bid	D	100%	100%	Avoid	Hemo: Not applicable CAPD: Not applicable CAVH: Not applicable

Chlorthalidone: Ineffective with low GFR. Binds to erythrocytes.

Furosemide: Ototoxicity alone or in combination with aminoglycosides.

Indapamide: Ototoxicity in combination with aminoglycosides. High doses effective in ESRD.

Metolazone: Ineffective in ESRD.

Piretanide: High doses effective in ESRD. Gynecomastia, impotence.

Spironolactone: High doses effective in ESRD. Ototoxicity. Active metabolites with long half-life. Hyperkalemia common when GFR < 30, especially in diabetics. Gynecomastia, hyperchloremic acidosis. Interferes with digoxin immunoassay.

Thiazides: Usually ineffective with GFR < 30 mL/min. Effective at low GFR in combination with loop diuretic. Hyperuricemia.

For definitions of the abbreviations used in the tables, see page 14.

Antihypertensive and Cardiovascular Agents (Continued)

Drug, Toxicity Notes	Percent Excreted Unchanged %	Half-Life (Normal/ ESRD) h	Plasma Protein Binding %	Volume of Distribution L/kg	Dose for Normal Renal Function	Method	GFR, mL/min >50	10-50	<10	Supplement for Dialysis
Torasemide	25	2-4/4-5	97-99	0.14-0.19	5 mg bid	D	100%	100%	100%	Hemo: None CAPD: None CAVH: No data
High doses effective in ESRD. Ototoxicity.										
Triamterene	5-10	2-12/10	40-70	2.2-3.7	25-50 mg bid	I	q12h	q12h	Avoid	Hemo: Not applicable CAPD: Not applicable CAVH: Not applicable
Hyperkalemia common when GFR < 30, especially in diabetics. Active metabolite with long half-life. Folic acid antagonist. Urolithiasis. Crystalluria in acid urine. Can cause acute renal failure.										

Miscellaneous Cardiac Drugs

Drug, Toxicity Notes	Percent Excreted Unchanged %	Half-Life (Normal/ ESRD) h	Plasma Protein Binding %	Volume of Distribution L/kg	Dose for Normal Renal Function	Method	GFR, mL/min >50	10-50	<10	Supplement for Dialysis
Amrinone	10-40	2.6-8.3/Unknown	20-40	1.3-1.6	5-10 µg/kg · min, daily dose < 10 mg/kg	D	100%	100%	50-75%	Hemo: No data CAPD: No data CAVH: No data
Thrombocytopenia. Gastrointestinal upset.										
Dobutamine	< 10	2 min/Unknown	Unknown	0.25	2.5-15 µg/kg · min	D	100%	100%	100%	Hemo: No data CAPD: No data CAVH: No data
Milrinone	80-85	1/1.5-3	Unknown	0.25-0.35	15-75 µg/kg iv as load, then 2.5-15 mg q6h po	D	100%	100%	50-75%	Hemo: No data CAPD: No data CAVH: No data

Nitrates

Isosorbide	10-20	0.15-0.5/4	72	1.5-4	10-20 mg tid	D	100%	100%	100%	Hemo: 10-20 mg CAPD: None CAVH: No data
	Active metabolites with long half-life.									
Nitroglycerine	< 1	2-4 min/ Unchanged	Unknown	2-3	Many methods and routes of dosing	D	100%	100%	100%	Hemo: No data CAPD: No data CAVH: No data

For definitions of the abbreviations used in the tables, see page 14.

Sedatives, Hypnotics, Drugs Used in Psychiatry

Psychotherapeutic drugs are commonly given to patients with renal disease to relieve anxiety and depression. Excessive sedation is the most frequent adverse effect in patients with renal insufficiency. Because malaise, somnolence, and encephalopathy are also common uremic symptoms, recognition of the adverse drug reactions can be delayed.

Benzodiazepines are often used to treat emotional stress associated with decreasing renal function in patients on dialysis, although the efficacy of chronic benzodiazepine treatment has been questioned. Members of this class are generally safer than other antianxiety agents and short-term administration is effective. Active polar metabolites of these compounds normally excreted by the kidneys are likely to accumulate in patients with renal impairment and produce enhanced, prolonged sedation. Diazepam, chlordiazepoxide, and flurazepam are examples of such compounds. Because of the potential for drug or metabolite accumulation, chronic use of these agents and others in this drug class should be discouraged in patients with decreased renal function.

Phenothiazines, used to treat major psychoses, and tricyclic antidepressants, used for severe depression in patients with renal disease, can also produce excessive sedation. Patients taking these drugs can also exhibit anticholinergic effects, orthostatic hypotension, confusion, and extrapyramidal symptoms.

Lithium carbonate has become an increasingly prescribed antidepressant. The drug is excreted by the kidney and has a narrow therapeutic range. Careful dose reduction and plasma lithium level monitoring is required in patients with impaired or unstable renal function. Hemodialysis has been used in cases of lithium overdose. Although lithium is effectively removed by dialysis, a rebound increase in plasma levels is common after hemodialysis, and repeated treatments may be required.

Sedatives, Hypnotics, Drugs Used in Psychiatry

Drug, Toxicity Notes	Percent Excreted Unchanged	Half-Life (Normal/ ESRD)	Plasma Protein Binding	Volume of Distribution	Dose for Normal Renal Function	Adjustment for Renal Failure Method	>50	10-50	<10	Supplement for Dialysis
	%	%	h	%	L/kg					
Antidepressants										
Amoxapine (Asendin)	Hepatic	8-30/Unknown	90	Unknown	75-200 mg/d	D	100%	100%	100%	Hemo: Unknown CAPD: Unknown CAVH: Unknown
T 1/2 of active metabolite is 30 hours.										
Bupropion	Hepatic	10-21/Unknown	82-88	27-36	100 mg q8h	D	100%	100%	100%	Hemo: Unknown CAPD: Unknown CAVH: Unknown
T 1/2 of active metabolite is 21 hours.										
Fluoxetine	Hepatic	24-72/Unchanged	94.5	20-42	20 mg/d	D	100%	100%	100%	Hemo: Unknown CAPD: Unknown CAVH: Unknown
T 1/2 of active metabolite is 7-9 days.										
Maprotiline	Hepatic	48/Unknown	Unknown	Unknown	75 mg/d	D	100%	100%	100%	Hemo: Unknown CAPD: Unknown CAVH: Unknown
Sertraline	Hepatic	24/Unknown	97	Unknown	50-200 mg/d	D	Unknown	Unknown	Unknown	Hemo: Unknown CAPD: Unknown CAVH: Unknown
Active metabolite.										

For definitions of the abbreviations used in the tables, see page 14.

57

Sedatives, Hypnotics, Drugs Used in Psychiatry (Continued)

Drug, Toxicity Notes	Percent Excreted Unchanged	Half-Life (Normal/ESRD)	Plasma Protein Binding	Volume of Distribution	Dose for Normal Renal Function	Adjustment for Renal Failure				Supplement for Dialysis
						Method	GFR, mL/min >50	10-50	<10	
	%	h	%	L/kg						
Trazodone	Renal	6-11/Unknown	Unknown	Unknown	150-400 mg/d	D	100%	Unknown	Unknown	Hemo: Unknown CAPD: Unknown CAVH: Unknown

Barbiturates

May cause excessive sedation, increase osteomalacia in ESRD. Charcoal hemoperfusion and hemodialysis more effective than peritoneal dialysis for overdose.

Drug, Toxicity Notes	Percent Excreted Unchanged	Half-Life (Normal/ESRD)	Plasma Protein Binding	Volume of Distribution	Dose for Normal Renal Function	Method	>50	10-50	<10	Supplement for Dialysis
Hexobarbital	Hepatic	3.5-4/Unknown	65	1.1	Unknown	D	100%	100%	100%	Hemo: None CAPD: Unknown CAVH: Unknown
Pentobarbital	Hepatic	18-48/Unchanged	60-70	1.0	30 mg tid-qid	D	100%	100%	100%	Hemo: None CAPD: Unknown CAVH: Unknown
Protein binding decreased in ESRD.										
Phenobarbital	Hepatic (renal)	60-150/117-160	40-60	0.7-1	50-100 mg bid-tid	I	q8-12h	q8-12h	q12-16h	Hemo: Dose after dialysis CAPD: 1/2 normal dose CAVH: None
Up to 50% unchanged drug excreted in urine with alkaline diuresis.										

Secobarbital	Hepatic	20-35/Unknown	44	1.5-2.5	30-50 mg tid-qid	D	100%	100%	100%	Hemo: None CAPD: None CAVH: Unknown
Thiopental	Hepatic	3.8/6-18	72-86	1-1.5	Anesthesia induction	D	100%	100%	75%	Hemo: Not applicable CAPD: Not applicable CAVH: Not applicable

Benzodiazepines

May cause excessive sedation and encephalopathy in ESRD.

Alprazolam	Hepatic	9.5-19/Unchanged	70-80	0.9-1.3	0.25-5.0 mg tid	D	100%	100%	100%	Hemo: None CAPD: Unknown CAVH: Unknown
Chlorazepate (Tranxene) Active metabolite.	Hepatic (renal)	39-85/36	Unknown	1.3	15-60 mg/d	D	100%	100%	100%	Hemo: Unknown CAPD: Unknown CAVH: Unknown
Chlordiazepoxide (Librium) Active metabolite.	Hepatic	5-30/Unchanged	94-97	0.3-0.5	15-100 mg/d	D	100%	100%	50%	Hemo: None CAPD: Unknown CAVH: Unknown
Clonazepam (Clonapin)	Hepatic	18-50/Unknown	47	1.5-4.5	1.5 mg/d	D	100%	100%	100%	Hemo: None CAPD: Unknown CAVH: Unknown

For definitions of the abbreviations used in the tables, see page 14.

Sedatives, Hypnotics, Drugs Used in Psychiatry (Continued)

Drug, Toxicity Notes	Percent Excreted Unchanged	Half-Life (Normal/ESRD)	Plasma Protein Binding	Volume of Distribution	Dose for Normal Renal Function	Adjustment for Renal Failure				Supplement for Dialysis
						Method	GFR, mL/min >50	10-50	<10	
	%	h	%	L/kg						
Diazepam (Valium)	Hepatic	20-90/Unchanged	94-98	0.7-3.4	5-40 mg/d	D	100%	100%	100%	Hemo: None CAPD: Unknown CAVH: Unknown
Active metabolite. Protein binding decreased in ESRD. Volume of distribution increased in ESRD.										
Estazolam	Hepatic	8-24/Unknown	93	Unknown	1 mg hs	D	100%	100%	100%	Hemo: Unknown CAPD: Unknown CAVH: Unknown
Flurazepam (Dalmane)	Hepatic	47-100/Unchanged	Unknown	3.4	15-30 mg hs	D	100%	100%	100%	Hemo: None CAPD: Unknown CAVH: Unknown
Active metabolite.										
Lorazepam (Ativan)	Hepatic	5-10/32-70	87	0.9-1.3	1-2 mg bid-tid	D	100%	100%	100%	Hemo: None CAPD: Unknown CAVH: Unknown
Midazolam	Hepatic	1.2-12.3/Unchanged	93-96	1.0-6.6	Individualized	D	100%	100%	50%	Hemo: Not applicable CAPD: Not applicable CAVH: Not applicable
Protein binding decreased in ESRD.										
Nitrazepam	Hepatic	18-36/Unknown	Unknown	Unknown	5-10 mg hs	D	100%	100%	100%	Hemo: Unknown CAPD: Unknown CAVH: Unknown

Oxazepam (Serax)	Hepatic	5-10/25-90	97	0.6-1.6	30-120 mg/d	D	100%	100%	100%	Hemo: None CAPD: Unknown CAVH: Unknown

Glucuronide metabolite increases in ESRD. Protein binding decreased and volume of distribution increased in ESRD.

Prazepam	Hepatic (renal)	36-200/36	Unknown	Unknown	20-60 mg hs	D	100%	100%	100%	Hemo: Unknown CAPD: Unknown CAVH: Unknown

Active metabolite.

Quazepam	Hepatic	20-40/Unknown	95	Unknown	15 mg hs	D	Unknown	Unknown	Unknown	Hemo: Unknown CAPD: Unknown CAVH: Unknown

Active metabolites.

Temazepam (Restoril)	Hepatic	4-10/Unknown	96	1.3-1.5	30 mg hs	D	100%	100%	100%	Hemo: None CAPD: None CAVH: Unknown

Protein binding decreased in renal disease.

Triazolam (Halcion)	Hepatic	2-4/Unchanged	85-95	Unknown	0.25-0.50 mg hs	D	100%	100%	100%	Hemo: None CAPD: None CAVH: Unknown

Protein binding correlates with alpha-1 acid glycoprotein concentration.

Benzodiazepine Antagonist

Flumazenil	Hepatic	0.7-1.3/Unknown	40-50	0.6-1.1	0.2 mg iv over 15 sec	D	100%	100%	100%	Hemo: None CAPD: Unknown CAVH: Unknown

For definitions of the abbreviations used in the tables, see page 14.

Sedatives, Hypnotics, Drugs Used in Psychiatry (Continued)

Drug, Toxicity Notes	Percent Excreted Unchanged	Half-Life (Normal/ESRD)	Plasma Protein Binding	Volume of Distribution	Dose for Normal Renal Function	Method	Adjustment for Renal Failure GFR, mL/min >50	10-50	<10	Supplement for Dialysis
	%	h	%	L/kg						
Miscellaneous Sedative Agents										
Buspirone	Hepatic	2-3/5.8	95	5	5 mg tid	D	100%	100%	100%	Hemo: None CAPD: Unknown CAVH: Unknown
Active metabolite accumulates.										
Chloral hydrate	Hepatic	7-14/Unknown	70-80	0.6	250 mg tid	D	100%	Avoid	Avoid	Hemo: None CAPD: Unknown CAVH: Unknown
Active metabolite. Excessive sedation.										
Ethchlorvynol	Hepatic	10-20	35-50	3-4	500 mg qhs	D	100%	Avoid	Avoid	Hemo: None CAPD: None CAVH: Unknown
Removed by hemoperfusion. Excessive sedation. Plasma levels rebound after dialysis.										
Haloperidol	Hepatic	10-19/Unknown	90-92	14-21	1-2 mg bid-tid	D	100%	100%	100%	Hemo: None CAPD: None CAVH: Unknown
Hypotension, excessive sedation.										
Lithium carbonate	Renal	14-28/40	None	0.5-0.9	0.9-1.2 g/d	D	100%	50-75%	25-50%	Hemo: Dose after dialysis CAPD: None CAVH: Unknown

Nephrotoxic. Nephrogenic diabetes inspidus. Nephrotic syndrome. Renal tubular acidosis. Interstitial fibrosis. Acute toxicity when serum levels > 1.2 mEq/L. Serum levels should be measured periodically 12 h after dose. T 1/2 does not reflect extensive tissue accumulation. Plasma levels rebound after dialysis. Toxicity enhanced by volume depletion, NSAIDs, diuretics.

Meprobamate	Hepatic (renal)	9-11/Unchanged	0-30	0.5-0.8	1200-1600 mg/d	I	q6h	q9-12h	q12-18h	Hemo: None CAPD: Unknown CAVH: Unknown

Excessive sedation. Excretion enhanced by forced diuresis.

Phenelzine	Hepatic	1.5-4/Unknown	Unknown	Unknown	45-75 mg/d	D	100%	100%	100%	Hemo: Unknown CAPD: Unknown CAVH: Unknown

Phenothiazines

Anticholinergic. Urinary retention. Orthostatic hypotension. Confusion. Extrapyramidal symptoms.

Chlorpromazine	Hepatic	11-42/Unchanged	91-99	8-160	300-800 mg/d	D	100%	100%	100%	Hemo: None CAPD: None CAVH: Unknown

Plasma levels rebound after oral dose.

Promethazine	Hepatic	9-12/Unknown	Unknown	Large	20-100 mg/d	D	100%	100%	100%	Hemo: Unknown CAPD: Unknown CAVH: Unknown

Excessive sedation.

For definitions of the abbreviations used in the tables, see page 14.

Sedatives, Hypnotics, Drugs Used in Psychiatry (Continued)

Drug, Toxicity Notes	Percent Excreted Unchanged		Half-Life (Normal/ ESRD)	Plasma Protein Binding	Volume of Distribution	Dose for Normal Renal Function	Adjustment for Renal Failure				Supplement for Dialysis
							Method	GFR, mL/min			
								>50	10-50	<10	
	%		h	%	L/kg						

Tricyclic Antidepressants

Anticholinergic. Urinary retention. Orthostatic hypotension. Confusion. Excessive sedation.

Drug, Toxicity Notes	Percent Excreted Unchanged		Half-Life (Normal/ESRD)	Plasma Protein Binding	Volume of Distribution	Dose for Normal Renal Function	Method	>50	10-50	<10	Supplement for Dialysis
Amitriptyline	Hepatic		24-40/Unchanged	96	6-36	25 mg tid	D	100%	100%	100%	Hemo: None / CAPD: None / CAVH: Unknown
Reduce dose in elderly.											
Clomipramine	Hepatic		19-37/Unknown	97	Unknown	100-250 mg/d	D	Unknown	Unknown	Unknown	Hemo: Unknown / CAPD: Unknown / CAVH: Unknown
Active metabolites.											
Desipramine	Hepatic		18-26/Unknown	92	10-50	100-200 mg/d	D	100%	100%	100%	Hemo: None / CAPD: None / CAVH: None
Active metabolites.											
Doxepin	Hepatic		8-25/10-30	95	9-33	25 mg tid	D	100%	100%	100%	Hemo: None / CAPD: None / CAVH: Unknown
Protein binding decreased in ESRD.											
Imipramine	Hepatic		12-24/Unknown	96	10-20	25 mg tid	D	100%	100%	100%	Hemo: None / CAPD: None / CAVH: None
Active metabolites.											

| Nortriptyline | Hepatic | 25-38/15-66 | 95 | 15-23 | 25 mg tid-qid | D | 100% | 100% | 100% | Hemo: None
CAPD: None
CAVH: Unknown |
| Protryptyline | Hepatic | 54-98/Unknown | 92 | 15-31 | 15-60 mg/d | D | 100% | 100% | 100% | Hemo: None
CAPD: None
CAVH: Unknown |

For definitions of the abbreviations used in the tables, see page 14.

Analgesics

Most commonly used analgesics are eliminated primarily by hepatic biotransformation and require little dose reduction for patients with renal insufficiency. Saturable, non-linear excretion complicates salicylate elimination kinetics. Because of the hemorrhagic diathesis in patients with severe renal failure and the variability of salicylate elimination, large doses of aspirin should be avoided in patients with severe renal failure. Narcotic analgesics produce sedation that may be more profound in patients with renal insufficiency. Doses of these drugs should be titrated carefully, and the minimum dose should be used for the shortest possible time.

Use of meperidine requires special care. The primary metabolite, normeperidine, has little analgesic effect, accumulates in patients with renal failure, and can decrease the seizure threshold. Although meperidine can be used in patients with severe renal failure, long-term therapy should be avoided.

Analgesics

Narcotics and Narcotic Antagonists

Drug, Toxicity Notes	Percent Excreted Unchanged	Half-Life (Normal/ ESRD)	Plasma Protein Binding	Volume of Distribution	Dose for Normal Renal Function	Adjustment for Renal Failure Method	>50	10-50	<10	Supplement for Dialysis
	%	h	%	L/kg						
Alfentanil	Hepatic	1-3/Unchanged	88-95	0.3-1	Anesthetic induction	D	100%	100%	100%	Hemo: Not applicable CAPD: Not applicable CAVH: Not applicable
Butorphanol	Hepatic	2-4/Unknown	80	9-11	2 mg q3-4h	D	100%	75%	50%	Hemo: Unknown CAPD: Unknown CAVH: Unknown
Codeine	Hepatic	2.5-3.5/Unknown	7	3-4	30-60 mg q4-6h	D	100%	75%	50%	Hemo: Unknown CAPD: Unknown CAVH: Unknown
Fentanyl	Hepatic	2-7/Unknown	80-84	2-4	Anesthetic induction	D	100%	75%	50%	Hemo: Not applicable CAPD: Not applicable CAVH: Not applicable

For definitions of the abbreviations used in the tables, see page 14.

67

Analgesics (Continued)

Drug, Toxicity Notes	Percent Excreted Unchanged %	Half-Life (Normal/ ESRD) h	Plasma Protein Binding %	Volume of Distribution L/kg	Dose for Normal Renal Function	Method	Adjustment for Renal Failure GFR, mL/min >50	10-50	<10	Supplement for Dialysis
Meperidine (Demerol)	Hepatic	2-7/7-32	70	4-5	50-100 mg q3-4h	D	100%	75%	50%	Hemo: None CAPD: None CAVH: Unknown
Normeperidine, an active metabolite, accumulates in ESRD and may cause seizures. Protein binding is reduced in ESRD. 20-25% excreted unchanged in acidic urine.										
Methadone	Hepatic	13-58/Unknown	60-90	3-6	2.5-10 mg q6-8h	D	100%	100%	50-75%	Hemo: None CAPD: None CAVH: Unknown
Fecal elimination is increased in ESRD.										
Morphine	Hepatic	1-4/Unchanged	20-30	3.5	20-25 mg q4h	D	100%	75%	50%	Hemo: None CAPD: Unknown CAVH: Unknown
Increased sensitivity to drug effect in ESRD.										
Naloxone	Hepatic	1-1.5/Unknown	54	3	2 mg iv	D	100%	100%	100%	Hemo: Not applicable CAPD: Not applicable CAVH: Not applicable
Pentazocine (Talwin)	Hepatic	2-5/Unknown	50-75	5	50 mg q4h	D	100%	75%	50%	Hemo: None CAPD: Unknown CAVH: Unknown
Propoxyphene (Darvon)	Hepatic	9-15/12-20	78	16	65 mg po tid-qid	D	100%	100%	Avoid	Hemo: None CAPD: None CAVH: Unknown
Active metabolite norpropoxyphene accumulates in ESRD.										

Drug	Route	t½ (Normal/ESRD)	% Protein Binding	Vd	Dose	D/I	GFR >50	GFR 10–50	GFR <10	Dialysis
Sufentanil	Hepatic	2-5/Unchanged	92	2-3	Anesthetic induction		100%	100%	100%	Hemo: Not applicable CAPD: Not applicable CAVH: Not applicable

Non-narcotic Drugs

Drug	Route	t½ (Normal/ESRD)	% Protein Binding	Vd	Dose	D/I	GFR >50	GFR 10–50	GFR <10	Dialysis
Acetaminophen	Hepatic	2/2	20-30	1-2	650 mg q4h	I	q4h	q6h	q8h	Hemo: None CAPD: None CAVH: Unknown
Acetylsalicylic acid (Aspirin)	Hepatic (renal)	2-3/Unchanged	80-90	0.1-0.2	650 mg q4h	I	q4h	q4-6h	Avoid	Hemo: Dose after dialysis CAPD: None CAVH: Unknown

Acetaminophen: Nephrotoxic in overdoses due to a reactive alkylating metabolite. Metabolites may accumulate in ESRD. Drug is major metabolite of phenacetin.

Acetylsalicylic acid: Nephrotoxic in high doses. May decrease GFR when renal blood flow is prostaglandin dependent. Excretion enhanced in alkaline urine. May add to uremic gastrointestinal and hematologic symptoms. Protein binding reduced in ESRD. 5% excreted unchanged in acidic urine, 85% in alkaline urine.

For definitions of the abbreviations used in the tables, see page 14.

Miscellaneous Agents

Anticonvulsants

Generalized major motor seizures occur in patients with uremia; phenytoin is one of the most frequently used drugs for such seizures. Phenytoin absorption is slow and erratic; hepatic metabolism is concentration dependent and saturable; and distribution and elimination vary. In addition, phenytoin protein binding is decreased and distribution volume is increased in renal failure. With any given total serum phenytoin level, the concentration of active, free drug will be higher in patients with uremia than in patients with normal renal function. Most clinical laboratories measure the total serum drug concentration, and thus a low total phenytoin level in a patient with renal failure should not necessarily be interpreted as subtherapeutic.

Physical findings such as nystagmus may be helpful in deciding not to increase the dose. Seizures are also a manifestation of phenytoin excess, and small dosage increases may result in disproportionately large increases in the serum drug level. Dose increments should be small, sufficient time should be allowed for the patient to reach steady-state drug levels, and measurements of free serum phenytoin concentration should be done frequently in patients with uremia who are not responding to therapy.

Nonsteroidal Anti-inflammatory Drugs

Adverse effects of nonsteroidal anti-inflammatory drugs can result from either the pharmacologic action of prostaglandin synthesis inhibition or direct hypersensitivity. Prostaglandins are important in maintaining renal vasodilation and ensuring adequate renal blood flow. Nonsteroidal anti-inflammatory drugs are potent inhibitors of renal prostaglandin synthesis, resulting in renal arteriolar constriction, decreased renal blood flow, and a reduced glomerular filtration rate.

Prostaglandins are also important for maintaining fluid and electrolyte homeostasis. Reduction in glomerular filtration allows increased tubular reabsorption. Decreased prostaglandin production increases tubular chloride reabsorption in Henle's loop and increases the effect of antidiuretic hormone on the distal tubule. These effects may lead to salt and water retention. Renin generation is also diminished. The resultant decrease in plasma aldosterone production can lead to potassium retention and hyperkalemia in patients with decreased renal function. Adverse effects of nonsteroidal anti-inflammatory drugs are more clinically apparent in patients with decreased effective circulating fluid volume. Thus, patients with congestive heart failure, chronic liver disease, chronic renal failure, dehydration, or hemorrhage are at increased risk for adverse effects.

Acute renal failure, characterized by proteinuria or the nephrotic syndrome, hematuria, pyuria, and histologic evidence of immune glomerular injury or interstitial nephritis, is consistent with a hypersensitivity reaction. Discontinuing treatment with the nonsteroidal anti-inflammatory agent results in the gradual disappearance of proteinuria and a return toward normal renal function.

Miscellaneous Agents

Drug, Toxicity Notes	Percent Excreted Unchanged	Half-Life (Normal/ ESRD)	Plasma Protein Binding	Volume of Distribution	Dose for Normal Renal Function	Adjustment for Renal Failure			Supplement for Dialysis
						Method	GFR, mL/min		
							>50	10-50	<10	
	%	h	%	L/kg					
Anticoagulants									
Alteplase (tissue-type plasminogen activator [tPa])	Unknown	0.5	Unknown	0.10	60 mg over 1 h, then 20 mg/h for 2 h	D	100%	100%	100%	Hemo: Unknown CAPD: Unknown CAVH: Unknown
Anistreplase	Unknown	1.2	Unknown	0.08	30 U over 2-5 min	D	100%	100%	100%	Hemo: Unknown CAPD: Unknown CAVH: Unknown
Dipyridamole	Unknown	12/Unknown	99	2.4	50 mg tid	D	100%	100%	100%	Hemo: Unknown CAPD: Unknown CAVH: Unknown
Heparin Half-life increases with dose.	None	0.3-2/Unchanged	> 90	0.06-0.1	75 U/kg load, then 0.5 U/kg · min	D	100%	100%	100%	Hemo: None CAPD: None CAVH: None

Drug					Dose	Method	>50	10-50	<10	Dialysis
Low-molecular-weight heparin	Unknown	2.2-6/3.6-5	Unknown	0.06-0.13	30-40 mg bid	D	100%	100%	50%	Hemo: Unknown CAPD: Unknown CAVH: Unknown
Iloprost	Unknown	0.3-0.5	Unknown	0.7	0.5-2 ng/kg · min for 5-12 h	D	100%	100%	50%	Hemo: Unknown CAPD: Unknown CAVH: Unknown
Indobufen	Unknown	6-7/27-33	> 99	0.18-0.21	100-200 mg bid	D	100%	50%	25%	Hemo: Unknown CAPD: Unknown CAVH: Unknown
Streptokinase	None	0.6-1.5/Unknown	Unknown	0.02-0.08	250 000 U loading dose, then 100 000 U/h	D	100%	100%	100%	Hemo: Not applicable CAPD: Not applicable CAVH: Not applicable
Sulfinpyrazone	25-50	2.2-5/Unchanged	> 95	0.06	200 mg bid	D	100%	100%	Avoid	Hemo: None CAPD: None CAVH: None
		Occasional acute renal failure. Uricosuric effect lost at low GFR.								
Sulotroban	52-62	0.7-3/9-39	Unknown	Unknown	Unknown	D	50%	30%	10%	Hemo: Unknown CAPD: Unknown CAVH: Unknown
Ticlopidine	2	24-33/Unknown	98	Unknown	250 mg bid	D	50%	100%	100%	Hemo: Unknown CAPD: Unknown CAVH: Unknown
Tranexamic acid	90	1.5/Unknown	3	Unknown	25 mg/kg tid-qid	D	50%	25%	10%	Hemo: Unknown CAPD: Unknown CAVH: Unknown

For definitions of the abbreviations used in the tables, see page 14.

Miscellaneous Agents (Continued)

Drug, Toxicity Notes	Percent Excreted Unchanged %	Half-Life (Normal/ESRD) h	Plasma Protein Binding %	Volume of Distribution L/kg	Dose for Normal Renal Function	Method	Adjustment for Renal Failure GFR, mL/min >50	10-50	<10	Supplement for Dialysis
Urokinase	Unknown	Unknown	Unknown	Unknown	4400 U/kg load, then 4400 U/kg · h	D	Unknown	Unknown	Unknown	Hemo: Unknown CAPD: Unknown CAVH: Unknown
Warfarin	None	35-45/Unchanged	99	0.15	10-15 mg load, then 2-10 mg/d	D	100%	100%	100%	Hemo: None CAPD: None CAVH: None
Follow prothrombin time. Decreased protein binding in uremia.										

Anticonvulsants

Monitor serum levels.

Drug, Toxicity Notes	Percent Excreted Unchanged %	Half-Life (Normal/ESRD) h	Plasma Protein Binding %	Volume of Distribution L/kg	Dose for Normal Renal Function	Method	Adjustment for Renal Failure GFR, mL/min >50	10-50	<10	Supplement for Dialysis
Carbamazepine	2-3	24 single dose; 4-6 chronic dosing	75	0.8-1.6	200 mg bid to 1200 mg/d	D	100%	100%	100%	Hemo: None CAPD: None CAVH: None
May cause inappropriate antidiuretic hormone secretion.										

Drug	Half-life (Normal/ESRD)	Protein binding (%)	Volume of distribution	Dose	Method	GFR >50	GFR 10-50	GFR <10	Supplement
Ethosuximide	17-40	35-55/Unchanged	10	0.6-0.9	500-1500 mg/d	D	100%	100%	100%	Hemo: None CAPD: Unknown CAVH: Unknown
Lamotrigine	<7	18-30/Unchanged	40-60	1.2	Unknown	D	100%	100%	100%	Hemo: None CAPD: Unknown CAVH: Unknown
Oxcarbazepine	<1	8-9/Unknown	40	0.7-0.8	200-400 mg tid	D	100%	100%	100%	Hemo: None CAPD: Unknown CAVH: Unknown
Phenytoin	2	24/Unchanged	90	1.0	1000 mg load, then 300-400 mg/d	D	100%	100%	100%	Hemo: None CAPD: None CAVH: None
Primidone	40	5-15/Unchanged	20-30	0.4-1.0	250-500 mg qid	I	q8h	q8-12h	q12-24h	Hemo: 1/3 dose CAPD: Unknown CAVH: Unknown
Sodium valproate	3-7	6-15/Unchanged	90	0.19-0.23	15-60 mg/kg · d	D	100%	100%	100%	Hemo: None CAPD: None CAVH: None
Trimethadione	None	12-24/Unknown	None	Unknown	300-600 mg tid-qid	I	q8h	q8-12h	q12-24h	Hemo: Unknown CAPD: Unknown CAVH: Unknown

Phenytoin: Measure free and bound levels. Protein binding decreased and distribution volume increased in renal failure. May cause interstitial nephritis. Saturable metabolism. folate deficiency.

Primidone: Partially converted to phenobarbital and other metabolites with long half-life. Excessive sedation. Nystagmus. Folate deficiency.

Sodium valproate: Decreased protein binding in uremia. Concurrent phenytoin, phenobarbital, and primidone shorten half-life.

Trimethadione: Active metabolites with long half-life. Nephrotic syndrome.

For definitions of the abbreviations used in the tables, see page 14.

Miscellaneous Agents (Continued)

Drug, Toxicity Notes	Percent Excreted Unchanged	Half-Life (Normal/ESRD)	Plasma Protein Binding	Volume of Distribution	Dose for Normal Renal Function	Adjustment for Renal Failure Method	GFR, mL/min >50	GFR, mL/min 10-50	GFR, mL/min <10	Supplement for Dialysis
	%	h	%	L/kg						
Vigabatrin	50-65	5-7/13-15	None	0.8	1-2 g bid	D	100%	50%	25%	Hemo: Unknown CAPD: Unknown CAVH: Unknown

Antihistamines

H-1 Antagonists

May cause excessive sedation.

Drug, Toxicity Notes	Percent Excreted Unchanged	Half-Life (Normal/ESRD)	Plasma Protein Binding	Volume of Distribution	Dose for Normal Renal Function	Adjustment for Renal Failure Method	GFR, mL/min >50	GFR, mL/min 10-50	GFR, mL/min <10	Supplement for Dialysis
Acrivastine	Unknown	1.4-2.1/Unknown	50	0.6-0.7	8 mg tid or qid	D	Unknown	Unknown	Unknown	Hemo: Unknown CAPD: Unknown CAVH: Unknown
Astemizole	None	20 d/Unchanged	97	Unknown	10 mg/d	D	100%	100%	100%	Hemo: Unknown CAPD: Unknown CAVH: Unknown

Brompheniramine	3	6/Unknown	Unknown	12	4 mg q4-6h	D	100%	100%	100%	Hemo: Unknown CAPD: Unknown CAVH: Unknown
Cetirizine	60-70	7-10/20	93	0.4-0.6	5-20 mg qd	D	100%	100%	30%	Hemo: None CAPD: Unknown CAVH: Unknown
Chlorpheniramine	20	14-24/Unknown	72	6-12	4 mg q4-6h	D	100%	100%	100%	Hemo: None CAPD: Unknown CAVH: Unknown
Diphenhydramine	2	3.4-9.3/Unknown	80	3.3-6.8	25 mg tid-qid	D	100%	100%	100%	Hemo: None CAPD: None CAVH: None
Anticholinergic effects may cause urine retention.										
Flunarizine	None	17-18 d/Unknown	99	43-78	10-20 mg/d	D	100%	100%	100%	Hemo: None CAPD: None CAVH: None
Hydroxyzine	None	14-20/Unknown	Unknown	19.5	50-100 mg qid	D	100%	Unknown	Unknown	Hemo: Unknown CAPD: Unknown CAVH: Unknown
Orphenadrine	8	16/Unknown	Unknown	Unknown	100 mg bid	D	100%	100%	100%	Hemo: Unknown CAPD: Unknown CAVH: Unknown
Active metabolite excreted by the kidney.										
Oxatomide	None	20/Unknown	91	Unknown	Unknown	D	100%	100%	100%	Hemo: None CAPD: None CAVH: None

For definitions of the abbreviations used in the tables, see page 14.

Miscellaneous Agents (Continued)

Drug, Toxicity Notes	Percent Excreted Unchanged %	Half-Life (Normal/ESRD) h	Plasma Protein Binding %	Volume of Distribution L/kg	Dose for Normal Renal Function	Method	Adjustment for Renal Failure GFR, mL/min >50	10-50	<10	Supplement for Dialysis
Promethazine	None	12/Unknown	93	13.5	12.5-25 mg qd-qid	D	100%	100%	100%	Hemo: None CAPD: None CAVH: None
Terfenadine	None	16-23/Unknown	97	Unknown	60 mg bid	D	100%	100%	100%	Hemo: None CAPD: None CAVH: None
Tripelennamine	Unknown	3-4.5/Unknown	Unknown	10	25-50 mg tid-qid	D	Unknown	Unknown	Unknown	Hemo: Unknown CAPD: Unknown CAVH: Unknown
Triprolidine	Unknown	5/Unknown	Unknown	Unknown	2.5 mg q4-6h	D	Unknown*	Unknown	Unknown	Hemo: Unknown CAPD: Unknown CAVH: Unknown

H-2 Antagonists

Cimetidine	50-70	1.5-2/5	20	0.8-1.3	400 mg bid or 400-800 mg qhs	D	100%	50%	25%	Hemo: None CAPD: None CAVH: Unknown

Increases serum creatinine and decreases creatinine clearance by inhibition of tubular creatinine secretion. Mental confusion in patients with renal or hepatic disease. Acute renal failure reported.

Drug									
Famotidine	65-80	2.5-4/12-19	15-22	0.8-1.4	20-40 mg qhs	D	50%	25%	10%	Hemo: None CAPD: None CAVH: None
Nizatidine	54-65	1.3-1.6/5.3-8.5	28-35	0.8-1.3	150-300 mg qhs	D	75%	50%	25%	Hemo: Unknown CAPD: Unknown CAVH: Unknown
Ranitidine	80	1.5-3/6-9	15	1.2-1.8	150-300 mg qhs	D	75%	50%	25%	Hemo: 1/2 dose CAPD: None CAVH: Unknown

Antineoplastic Agents

Most agents in this group are myelosuppressive and may aggravate uremic predisposition to hemorrhage and infection.

Drug									
Azathioprine	<2	0.16-1/Increased	20	0.55-0.8	1.5-2.5 mg/kg · d	D	100%	75%	50%	Hemo: Yes CAPD: Unknown CAVH: Unknown

Mercaptopurine is active metabolite.

Bleomycin	60	9/20	Unknown	0.3	10-20 U/m^2	D	100%	75%	50%	Hemo: None CAPD: Unknown CAVH: Unknown

Drug accumulation predisposes to pulmonary fibrosis. Hypertension and dysuria.

Busulfan	0.5-3	2.5-3.4/Unknown	3-15	1	4-8 mg/d	D	100%	100%	100%	Hemo: Unknown CAPD: Unknown CAVH: Unknown

May cause hemorrhagic cystitis.

For definitions of the abbreviations used in the tables, see page 14.

Miscellaneous Agents (Continued)

Drug, Toxicity Notes	Percent Excreted Unchanged %	Half-Life (Normal/ ESRD) h	Plasma Protein Binding %	Volume of Distribution L/kg	Dose for Normal Renal Function	Adjustment for Renal Failure Method	>50	GFR, mL/min 10-50	<10	Supplement for Dialysis
Carboplatin	50-75	6/Increased	15-24	0.23-0.28	360 mg/m²	D	100%	50%	25%	Hemo: Unknown CAPD: Unknown CAVH: Unknown
Carmustine	Unknown	1.5/Unknown	Unknown	3.3	150-200 mg/m²	D	Unknown	Unknown	Unknown	Hemo: Unknown CAPD: Unknown CAVH: Unknown
Chlorambucil	Unknown	1/Unknown	Unknown	0.86	0.1 mg/kg · d	D	Unknown	Unknown	Unknown	Hemo: Unknown CAPD: Unknown CAVH: Unknown
Cisplatin	27-45	0.3-0.5/Unknown	90	0.5	20-50 mg/m² · d	D	100%	75%	50%	Hemo: Yes CAPD: Unknown CAVH: Unknown
Nephrotoxic. Toxicity reduced by pretreatment hydration. Renal Mg⁺⁺ wasting.										
Cyclophosphamide	10-15	4-7.5/10	14	0.62	1-5 mg/kg · d	D	100%	100%	75%	Hemo: 1/2 dose CAPD: Unknown CAVH: Unknown
Hemorrhagic cystitis. Bladder fibrosis and bladder cancer. SIADH.										
Cytarabine	6	0.5-3/Unchanged	13	2.6	100-200 mg/m²	D	100%	100%	100%	Hemo: Unknown CAPD: Unknown CAVH: Unknown

Drug					Dose		GFR >50	GFR 10–50	GFR <10	Dialysis
Daunorubicin	None	18-27/Unknown	Unknown	Unknown	30-45 mg/m^2	D	100%	100%	100%	Hemo: Unknown CAPD: Unknown CAVH: Unknown
Doxorubicin	< 15	35/Unchanged	80-85	21.5	60-75 mg/m^2 · d	D	100%	100%	100%	Hemo: None CAPD: Unknown CAVH: Unknown
Etoposide	20-60	4-8/19	74-94	0.17-0.5	35-100 mg/m^2 · d	D	100%	75%	50%	Hemo: None CAPD: Unknown CAVH: Unknown
Fluorouracil	< 5	0.1/Unchanged	10	0.25-0.5	12 mg/kg · d	D	100%	100%	100%	Hemo: Yes CAPD: Unknown CAVH: Unknown
Hydroxyurea	Substantial	Unknown	Unknown	0.5	20-30 mg/kg · d	D	100%	50%	20%	Hemo: Unknown CAPD: Unknown CAVH: Unknown
Ifosfamide	15	4-10/Unknown	Unknown	0.4-0.64	1.2 g/m^2	D	100%	100%	100%	Hemo: Unknown CAPD: Unknown CAVH: Unknown
Melphalan	12	1.1-1.4/4-6	90	0.6-0.75	6 mg/d	D	100%	75%	50%	Hemo: Unknown CAPD: Unknown CAVH: Unknown
Methotrexate	80-90	8-12/Increased	45-50	0.76	5-10 mg/wk for RA; 15 mg/d to 12 g/m^2 for cancer	D	100%	50%	Avoid	Hemo: None CAPD: None CAVH: Unknown

Doxorubicin: Acute renal failure and nephrotic syndrome.

Methotrexate: Nephrotoxicity prevented by urinary alkalinization and forced diuresis.

For definitions of the abbreviations used in the tables, see page 14.

Miscellaneous Agents (Continued)

Drug, Toxicity Notes	Percent Excreted Unchanged %	Half-Life (Normal/ESRD) h	Plasma Protein Binding %	Volume of Distribution L/kg	Dose for Normal Renal Function	Method	Adjustment for Renal Failure GFR, mL/min >50	10-50	<10	Supplement for Dialysis
Mitomycin C	Unknown	0.5-1/Unknown	Unknown	0.5	20 mg/m² q6-8 wk	D	100%	100%	75%	Hemo: Unknown CAPD: Unknown CAVH: Unknown
Nitrosoureas	Substantial	Short/Unknown	Unknown	Unknown	Varies	D	100%	75%	25-50%	Hemo: None CAPD: Unknown CAVH: Unknown
Plicamycin	Substantial	2/Unknown	Low	Unknown	25-30 µg/kg · d	D	100%	75%	50%	Hemo: Unknown CAPD: Unknown CAVH: Unknown
Streptozotocin	None	0.25/Unknown	Unknown	0.5	500 mg/m² · d	D	100%	75%	50%	Hemo: Unknown CAPD: Unknown CAVH: Unknown
Tamoxifen	None	18/Unknown	> 98	20	10-20 mg bid	D	100%	100%	100%	Hemo: Unknown CAPD: Unknown CAVH: Unknown

Mitomycin C: Nephrotoxicity. Hemolytic uremic syndrome.

Nitrosoureas: Prototype methyl CCNU. Metabolites with variable T 1/2. Irreversible toxicity at dose > 1500 mg/m².

Plicamycin: Cumulative nephrotoxicity. Acute renal failure. Decrease Ca⁺⁺, K⁺, PO₄.

Tamoxifen: Nephrotoxic. Proteinuria. Low PO₄. Renal tubular acidosis.

Drug										Dialysis
Teniposide	4-14	6-10/Unknown	99	0.2-0.7	50-250 mg/m^2	D	100%	100%	100%	Hemo: None / CAPD: None / CAVH: None
Vinblastine	None	1-1.5/Unknown	75	13-40	3.7 mg/m^2	D	100%	100%	100%	Hemo: Unknown / CAPD: Unknown / CAVH: Unknown

Vinca alkaloids may cause SIADH. Volume of distribution increases with time due to avid tissue binding.

Drug										Dialysis
Vincristine	12	1-2.5/Unknown	75	5-11	1.4 mg/m^2	D	100%	100%	100%	Hemo: Unknown / CAPD: Unknown / CAVH: Unknown

Antiparkinson Agents

Require careful titration of dose according to clinical response.

Drug										Dialysis
Bromocriptine	None	3/Unknown	90-96	Unknown	1.25 mg bid	D	100%	100%	100%	Hemo: Unknown / CAPD: Unknown / CAVH: Unknown

Orthostatic hypotension. Digital vasospasm.

Drug										Dialysis
Carbidopa	30	2/Unknown	Unknown	Unknown	1 tab tid to 6 tabs daily	D	100%	100%	100%	Hemo: Unknown / CAPD: Unknown / CAVH: Unknown
Levodopa	None	0.8-1.6/Unknown	5-8	0.9-1.6	250-500 mg bid to 8 g/d	D	100%	100%	100%	Hemo: Unknown / CAPD: Unknown / CAVH: Unknown

Active and inactive metabolites excreted in urine. Active metabolites with long T 1/2.

For definitions of the abbreviations used in the tables, see page 14.

Miscellaneous Agents *(Continued)*

Drug, Toxicity Notes	Percent Excreted Unchanged	Half-Life (Normal/ESRD)	Plasma Protein Binding	Volume of Distribution	Dose for Normal Renal Function	Adjustment for Renal Failure				Supplement for Dialysis
						Method	GFR, *mL/min*			
							>50	10-50	<10	
	%	h	%	L/kg						
Trihexyphenidyl	Unknown	10/Unknown	Unknown	Unknown	1-2 mg/d to 6-10 mg/d	D	Unknown	Unknown	Unknown	Hemo: Unknown CAPD: Unknown CAVH: Unknown
Anticholinergic effects may cause urinary retention.										
Antithyroid Drugs										
Methimazole	7	3-6/Unchanged	None	0.6	5-20 mg tid	D	100%	100%	100%	Hemo: Unknown CAPD: Unknown CAVH: Unknown
Propylthiouracil	<10	1-2/Unchanged	80	0.3-0.4	100 mg tid	D	100%	100%	100%	Hemo: Unknown CAPD: Unknown CAVH: Unknown

						75%	50%	25%	
Allopurinol	30	2-8/Unchanged	< 5	0.5	300 mg/d	D	75%	50%	25%	Hemo: 1/2 dose CAPD: Unknown CAVH: Unknown

Interstitial nephritis. Rare xanthine stones. Renal excretion of active metabolite with T 1/2 of 25 hours in normal renal function; one week in patients with ESRD. Exfoliative dermatitis.

Auranofin	50	70-80 d/Unknown	60	Unknown	6 mg/d	D	50%	Avoid	Avoid	Hemo: None CAPD: None CAVH: None

Rarely nephrotoxic. Proteinuria and nephrotic syndrome common.

Colchicine	5-17	19/40	31	2.2	Acute: 2 mg then 0.5 mg q6h Chronic: 0.5-1 mg/d	D	100%	100%	50%	Hemo: None CAPD: Unknown CAVH: Unknown

Avoid prolonged use if GFR < 50 mL/min.

Gold sodium thiomalate	60-90	250 d/Unknown	95	5-9	25-50 mg	D	50%	Avoid	Avoid	Hemo: None CAPD: None CAVH: None

Nephrotoxic. Proteinuria, membranous nephritis.

Penicillamine	40	1.5-3/Increased	80	Unknown	250-1000 mg/d	D	100%	Avoid	Avoid	Hemo: 1/3 dose CAPD: Unknown CAVH: Unknown

Reversible nephrotic syndrome.

Probenecid	< 2	5-8/Unchanged	85-95	0.15	500 mg bid	D	100%	Avoid	Avoid	Hemo: Unknown CAPD: Unknown CAVH: Unknown

Ineffective at decreased GFR.

For definitions of the abbreviations used in the tables, see page 14.

Miscellaneous Agents (Continued)

Drug, Toxicity Notes	Percent Excreted Unchanged	Half-Life (Normal/ ESRD)	Plasma Protein Binding	Volume of Distribution	Dose for Normal Renal Function	Method	Adjustment for Renal Failure GFR, mL/min >50	Adjustment for Renal Failure GFR, mL/min 10-50	Adjustment for Renal Failure GFR, mL/min <10	Supplement for Dialysis
	%	h	%	L/kg						

Nonsteroidal Anti-inflammatory Drugs

May decrease renal function. Decrease platelet aggregation. Nephrotic syndrome. Interstitial nephritis. Hyperkalemia. Sodium retention.

Drug	Percent Excreted Unchanged	Half-Life	Plasma Protein Binding	Volume of Distribution	Dose for Normal Renal Function	Method	>50	10-50	<10	Supplement for Dialysis
Diclofenac	<1	1-2/Unchanged	>99	0.12-0.17	25-75 mg bid	D	100%	100%	100%	Hemo: None CAPD: None CAVH: None
Diflunisal	<3	5-20/62	>99	0.10-0.13	250-500 mg bid	D	100%	50%	50%	Hemo: None CAPD: None CAVH: None
Etodolac	Negligible	5-7/Unchanged	>99	0.4	200 mg bid	D	100%	100%	100%	Hemo: None CAPD: None CAVH: None
Fenoprofen	30	2-3/Unchanged	>99	0.10	300-600 mg qid	D	100%	100%	100%	Hemo: None CAPD: None CAVH: None
Flurbiprofen	<15	3-5/Unchanged	99	0.10	100 mg bid-tid	D	100%	100%	100%	Hemo: None CAPD: None CAVH: None

Ibuprofen	1	2-3.2/Unchanged	99	0.15-0.17	800 mg tid	D	100%	100%	100%	Hemo: None CAPD: None CAVH: None
Indomethacin	30	4-12/Unchanged	99	0.12	25-50 mg tid	D	100%	100%	100%	Hemo: None CAPD: None CAVH: None
Isoxicam	Unknown	10-54/Unchanged	Unknown	0.20	200 mg/d	D	100%	100%	100%	Hemo: None CAPD: None CAVH: None
Ketoprofen	<1	1.5-4/Unchanged	99	0.11	25-75 mg tid	D	100%	100%	100%	Hemo: None CAPD: None CAVH: None
Ketorolac	5-10	4-6/10	>99	0.13-0.25	30-60 mg loading dose, then 15-30 mg q6h	D	100%	50%	50%	Hemo: None CAPD: None CAVH: None
Meclofenamic acid	2-4	3/Unchanged	>99	Unknown	50-100 mg tid-qid	D	100%	100%	100%	Hemo: None CAPD: None CAVH: None
Mefenamic acid	<6	3-4/Unchanged	Unknown	Unknown	250 mg qid	D	100%	100%	100%	Hemo: None CAPD: None CAVH: None
Nabumetone	<1	24/Unchanged	>99	0.11	1000-2000 mg/d	D	100%	100%	100%	Hemo: None CAPD: None CAVH: None

For definitions of the abbreviations used in the tables, see page 14.

Miscellaneous Agents (Continued)

Drug, Toxicity Notes	Percent Excreted Unchanged	Half-Life (Normal/ ESRD)	Plasma Protein Binding	Volume of Distribution	Dose for Normal Renal Function	Adjustment for Renal Failure				Supplement for Dialysis
						Method	GFR, mL/min			
							>50	10-50	<10	
	%	h	%	L/kg						
Naproxen	<1	12-15/Unchanged	99	0.10	500 mg bid	D	100%	100%	100%	Hemo: None CAPD: None CAVH: None
Oxaproxin	<1	50-60/Unchanged	>99	0.20	1200 mg/d	D	100%	100%	100%	Hemo: None CAPD: None CAVH: None
Phenylbutazone	1	50-100/Unchanged	99	0.09-0.17	100 mg tid-qid	D	100%	100%	100%	Hemo: None CAPD: None CAVH: None
Piroxicam	10	45-55/Unchanged	>99	0.12-0.15	20 mg/d	D	100%	100%	100%	Hemo: None CAPD: None CAVH: None
Sulindac	7	8-16/Unchanged	95	Unknown	200 mg bid	D	100%	100%	100%	Hemo: None CAPD: None CAVH: None
Tolmetin	15	1-1.5/Unchanged	>99	0.10-0.14	400 mg tid	D	100%	100%	100%	Hemo: None CAPD: None CAVH: None

. Active sulfide metabolite.

Bronchodilators

Drug	% Protein binding	Half-life (normal/ESRD)	Vd	Dose	Method	GFR >50	GFR 10-50	GFR <10	Supplement
Albuterol	51-64	2-4/4	7	2.0-2.5	2-4 mg tid to qid	D	100%	75%	50%	Hemo: Unknown CAPD: Unknown CAVH: Unknown
Dyphylline	85	1.8-2.3/12	<3	0.8	15 mg/kg · d	D	75%	50%	25%	Hemo: 1/3 dose CAPD: Unknown CAVH: Unknown
Ipratropium	Unknown	1.6/Unknown	Unknown	4.6	2 inhalations qid	D	100%	100%	100%	Hemo: None CAPD: None CAVH: None
Metaproterenol	Unknown	2-6/Unknown	10	7.6	2-3 inhalations q3-4h	D	100%	100%	100%	Hemo: Unknown CAPD: Unknown CAVH: Unknown
Terbutaline	55-60	3/Unknown	15-25	0.9-1.5	2.5-5 mg tid	D	100%	50%	Avoid	Hemo: Unknown CAPD: Unknown CAVH: Unknown

Large first dose effect. Parenteral doses should be avoided in ESRD. Oral doses unchanged.

Drug	% Protein binding	Half-life (normal/ESRD)	Vd	Dose	Method	GFR >50	GFR 10-50	GFR <10	Supplement
Theophylline	None	4-12/Unchanged	55	0.4-0.7	6 mg/kg load, then 9 mg/kg · d	D	100%	100%	100%	Hemo: 1/2 dose CAPD: Unknown CAVH: Unknown

May exacerbate uremic gastrointestinal symptoms.

For definitions of the abbreviations used in the tables, see page 14.

Miscellaneous Agents *(Continued)*

Drug, Toxicity Notes	Percent Excreted Unchanged	Half-Life (Normal/ ESRD)	Plasma Protein Binding	Volume of Distribution	Dose for Normal Renal Function	Adjustment for Renal Failure Method	>50	10-50	<10	Supplement for Dialysis
	%	h	%	L/kg				GFR, mL/min		

Corticosteroids

May aggravate azotemia, Na⁺ retention, glucose intolerance, and hypertension.

Drug	%	h	%	L/kg	Dose	Method	>50	10-50	<10	Supplement for Dialysis
Betamethasone	5	5.5/Unknown	65	1.4	0.5-9 mg/d	D	100%	100%	100%	Hemo: Unknown CAPD: Unknown CAVH: Unknown
Budesonide	None	2-2.7/Unknown	88	4.3	Unknown	D	100%	100%	100%	Hemo: Unknown CAPD: Unknown CAVH: Unknown
Cortisone	None	0.5-2/3.5	90	Unknown	25-500 mg/d	D	100%	100%	100%	Hemo: None CAPD: Unknown CAVH: Unknown
Dexamethasone	8	3-4/Unknown	70	0.8-1.0	0.75-9 mg/d	D	100%	100%	100%	Hemo: Unknown CAPD: Unknown CAVH: Unknown
Hydrocortisone	None	1.5-2/Unknown	Unknown	Unknown	20-500 mg/d	D	100%	100%	100%	Hemo: Unknown CAPD: Unknown CAVH: Unknown

Drug	% Protein Binding	Half-life (Normal/ESRD)			Dose	Method	>50	10–50	<10	Dialysis
Methylprednisolone	<10	1.9-6/Unchanged	40-60	1.2-1.5	4-48 mg/d	D	100%	100%	100%	Hemo: Yes / CAPD: Unknown / CAVH: Unknown
Prednisolone	34	2.5-3.5/Unchanged	Saturable	2.2	5-60 mg/d	D	100%	100%	100%	Hemo: Yes / CAPD: Unknown / CAVH: Unknown
Prednisone	34	2.5-3.5/Unchanged	Saturable	2.2	5-60 mg/d	D	100%	100%	100%	Hemo: None / CAPD: Unknown / CAVH: Unknown
Triamcinolone	Unknown	1.9-6/Unchanged	Unknown	1.4-2.1	4-48 mg/d	D	100%	100%	100%	Hemo: Unknown / CAPD: Unknown / CAVH: Unknown

Hypoglycemic Agents

Drug	% Protein Binding	Half-life (Normal/ESRD)			Dose	Method	>50	10–50	<10	Dialysis
Acetohexamide	None	1-1.3/Unchanged	65-90	0.21	250-1500 mg/d	I	Avoid	Avoid	Avoid	Hemo: Unknown / CAPD: None / CAVH: Unknown

Has diuretic effect. May falsely elevate serum creatinine. Active metabolite has T 1/2 of 5-8 hours in healthy subjects and is eliminated by the kidney. Prolonged hypoglycemia in azotemic patients.

Drug	% Protein Binding	Half-life (Normal/ESRD)			Dose	Method	>50	10–50	<10	Dialysis
Chlorpropamide	47	24-48/50-200	88-96	0.09-0.27	100-500 mg/d	D	50%	Avoid	Avoid	Hemo: Unknown / CAPD: None / CAVH: Unknown

Impairs water excretion. Prolonged hypoglycemia in azotemic patients.

For definitions of the abbreviations used in the tables, see page 14.

Miscellaneous Agents (Continued)

Drug, Toxicity Notes	Percent Excreted Unchanged	Half-Life (Normal/ ESRD)	Plasma Protein Binding	Volume of Distribution	Dose for Normal Renal Function	Adjustment for Renal Failure				Supplement for Dialysis
						Method	GFR, mL/min			
							>50	10-50	<10	
	%	h	%	L/kg						
Glibornuride	Unknown	5-12/Unknown	95	0.25	12.5-100 mg/d	D	Unknown	Unknown	Unknown	Hemo: Unknown CAPD: Unknown CAVH: Unknown
Gliclazide	< 20	8-11/Unknown	85-95	0.24	80-320 mg/d	D	Unknown	Unknown	Unknown	Hemo: Unknown CAPD: Unknown CAVH: Unknown
Glipizide	4.5-7	3-7/Unknown	97	0.13-0.16	2.5-15 mg/d	D	100%	100%	100%	Hemo: Unknown CAPD: Unknown CAVH: Unknown
Glyburide	50	1.4-2.9/Unknown	99	0.16-0.3	1.25-20 mg/d	D	Unknown	Avoid	Avoid	Hemo: None CAPD: None CAVH: None
Insulin	None	2-4/Increased	5	0.15	Variable	D	100%	75%	50%	Hemo: None CAPD: None CAVH: None
Tolazamide	7	4-7/Unknown	94	Unknown	100-250 mg/d	D	100%	100%	100%	Hemo: Unknown CAPD: Unknown CAVH: Unknown

Renal metabolism of insulin decreases with azotemia.

Has diuretic effect.

Drug	% Excreted	Half-life (Normal/ESRD)	Protein Binding	Vd	Dose	Method	GFR >50	GFR 10-50	GFR <10	Supplement
Tolbutamide	None	4-6/Unchanged	95-97	0.10-0.15	1-2 g/d	D	100%	100%	100%	Hemo: None CAPD: None CAVH: None

May impair water excretion.

Hypolipidemic Agents

Drug	% Excreted	Half-life (Normal/ESRD)	Protein Binding	Vd	Dose	Method	GFR >50	GFR 10-50	GFR <10	Supplement
Bezafibrate	35-40	2.1/7.8	95	0.24-0.35	Unknown	D	70%	50%	25%	Hemo: Unknown CAPD: Unknown CAVH: Unknown
Cholestyramine	None	Not absorbed	None	None	4 g q4-6h	D	100%	100%	100%	Hemo: None CAPD: None CAVH: None
Clofibrate	40-70	15-17.5/30-110	92-97	0.14	500-1000 mg bid	I	q6-12h	q12-18h	Avoid	Hemo: None CAPD: Unknown CAVH: Unknown
Colestipol	None	Not absorbed	None	None	13-30 g/d	D	100%	100%	100%	Hemo: None CAPD: None CAVH: None
Fluvastatin	<1	0.5-1/Unknown	Unknown	0.42	2-10 mg/d	D	100%	100%	100%	Hemo: Unknown CAPD: Unknown CAVH: Unknown
Gemfibrozil	None	7.6/Unchanged	97-99	Unknown	600 mg bid	D	100%	100%	100%	Hemo: None CAPD: Unknown CAVH: Unknown

Cholestyramine: Hyperchloremic acidosis.

Clofibrate: Impairs water excretion. Myositis.

Colestipol: Hyperchloremic acidosis.

For definitions of the abbreviations used in the tables, see page 14.

93

Miscellaneous Agents (Continued)

Drug, Toxicity Notes	Percent Excreted Unchanged	Half-Life (Normal/ESRD)	Plasma Protein Binding	Volume of Distribution	Dose for Normal Renal Function	Method	Adjustment for Renal Failure GFR, mL/min >50	10-50	<10	Supplement for Dialysis
	%	h	%	L/kg						
Lovastatin	None	1.1-1.7/Unchanged	> 95	Unknown	20-80 mg/d	D	100%	100%	100%	Hemo: Unknown CAPD: Unknown CAVH: Unknown
Nicotinic acid	None	0.5-1/Unknown	Unknown	Unknown	1-2 g tid	D	100%	50%	25%	Hemo: Unknown CAPD: Unknown CAVH: Unknown
	Toxic reactions frequent in ESRD. Aspirin may attenuate flushing.									
Pravastatin	47	0.8-3.2/Unchanged	45	0.9	10-40 mg/d	D	100%	100%	100%	Hemo: Unknown CAPD: Unknown CAVH: Unknown
Probucol	< 2	23-47 d/Unknown	Unknown	Unknown	500 mg bid	D	100%	100%	100%	Hemo: Unknown CAPD: Unknown CAVH: Unknown
Simvastatin	< 0.5	Unknown	> 95	Unknown	5-40 mg/d	D	100%	100%	100%	Hemo: Unknown CAPD: Unknown CAVH: Unknown

For definitions of the abbreviations used in the tables, see page 14.

Miscellaneous Drugs

Drug	% Excreted Unchanged	Half-life Normal/ESRD	Protein Binding %	Vd	Dose	Method	>50	10-50	<10	Supplement
Acetohydroxamic acid	Substantial	3.5-5/15-23	Unknown	Unknown	10-15 mg/kg · d	D	100%	100%	Avoid	Hemo: Unknown / CAPD: Unknown / CAVH: Unknown
May accumulate in ESRD.										
Clodronate	70-90	13/Increased	36	0.25	3-10 mg/kg	D	Unknown	Unknown	Avoid	Hemo: Unknown / CAPD: Unknown / CAVH: Unknown
Hyperchloremic acidosis.										
Cyclosporine	< 1	3-16/Unchanged	96-99	3.5-7.4	3-10 mg/kg · d	D	100%	100%	100%	Hemo: None / CAPD: None / CAVH: Unknown
Nephrotoxic. Hypertension, seizures, tremor. Inhibitors of hepatic metabolism increase blood concentration.										
Desferoxamine	30-35	6/Unknown	Unknown	2-2.5	Acute: 1 g then 0.5 g q4-12h; Chronic: 0.5-1 g/d	D	100%	100%	50%	Hemo: Unknown / CAPD: Unknown / CAVH: Unknown
Metoclopramide	10-22	2.5-4/14-15	40	2-3.4	10-15 mg qid	D	100%	75%	50%	Hemo: None / CAPD: Unknown / CAVH: Unknown
Extrapyramidal side effects common in ESRD.										
N-Acetylcysteine	30	2.3-6/Unknown	50	0.33-0.47	140 mg/kg load, then 70 mg/kg q4h for 17 doses	D	100%	100%	75%	Hemo: Unknown / CAPD: Unknown / CAVH: Unknown
Pentoxifylline	None	0.8/Unchanged	None	2.4-4.2	400 mg tid	D	100%	100%	100%	Hemo: Unknown / CAPD: Unknown / CAVH: Unknown

For definitions of the abbreviations used in the tables, see page 14.

Miscellaneous Agents (Continued)

Drug, Toxicity Notes	Percent Excreted Unchanged	Half-Life (Normal/ ESRD)	Plasma Protein Binding	Volume of Distribution	Dose for Normal Renal Function	Adjustment for Renal Failure Method	Adjustment for Renal Failure GFR, mL/min >50	Adjustment for Renal Failure GFR, mL/min 10-50	Adjustment for Renal Failure GFR, mL/min <10	Supplement for Dialysis
	%	h	%	L/kg						
Neuromuscular Agents										
Alcuronium	80-85	3-3.5/16	40	0.28-0.36	Unknown	D	Avoid	Avoid	Avoid	Hemo: Unknown CAPD: Unknown CAVH: Unknown
Alfentanil	<1	1.4-2/Unchanged	88-95	0.3-1.0	8-245 μg/kg load, then 0.5-3 μg/kg · min	D	100%	100%	100%	Hemo: Unknown CAPD: Unknown CAVH: Unknown
Atracurium	None	0.3-0.4/Unchanged	82	0.15-0.18	0.4-0.5 mg/kg load, then 0.08-0.1 mg/kg q15-25 min	D	100%	100%	100%	Hemo: Unknown CAPD: Unknown CAVH: Unknown
Doxacurium	24-38	1.2-1.6/3.7	28-34	0.12-0.22	0.025-0.05 mg/kg	D	100%	50%	50%	Hemo: Unknown CAPD: Unknown CAVH: Unknown
Etomidate	2	4-5/Unchanged	75	2-4.5	0.2-0.6 mg/kg	D	100%	100%	100%	Hemo: Unknown CAPD: Unknown CAVH: Unknown

Drug					Dose					Dialysis
Fazadinium	None	1/Unchanged	17	0.18-0.23	1-2 mg/kg	D	100%	100%	100%	Hemo: Unknown CAPD: Unknown CAVH: Unknown
Fentanyl	6-8	2.5-3.5/Unchanged	79-87	2-5	0.002-0.05 mg/kg	D	100%	100%	100%	Hemo: Unknown CAPD: Unknown CAVH: Unknown
Gallamine	85-100	2.3-2.7/6-20	30-70	0.21-0.24	0.5-1.5 mg/kg	D	75%	Avoid	Avoid	Hemo: Not applicable CAPD: Not applicable CAVH: Not applicable

Recurarization may occur up to 24 hours after dose. If blockade not responsive to neostigmine, dialysis may be useful.

Drug					Dose					Dialysis
Ketamine	2-3	2-3.5/Unchanged	Unknown	1.8-3.1	1-4.5 mg/kg	D	100%	100%	100%	Hemo: Unknown CAPD: Unknown CAVH: Unknown
Metocurine	45-60	3.5-5.8/11.3	70	0.42-0.57	0.2-0.4 mg/kg	D	75%	50%	50%	Hemo: Unknown CAPD: Unknown CAVH: Unknown
Neostigmine	67	1.3/3.0	None	0.5-1.0	15-375 mg/d	D	100%	50%	25%	Hemo: Unknown CAPD: Unknown CAVH: Unknown
Pancuronium	30-40	1.7-2.2/4.3-8.2	70-85	0.15-0.38	0.04-0.1 mg/kg	D	100%	50%	Avoid	Hemo: Unknown CAPD: Unknown CAVH: Unknown

Recurarization may occur up to 24 hours after dose.

Drug					Dose					Dialysis
Pipecuronium	Unknown	2.3/4.4	Unknown	0.31	100 µg/kg	D	100%	50%	25%	Hemo: Unknown CAPD: Unknown CAVH: Unknown

For definitions of the abbreviations used in the tables, see page 14.

Miscellaneous Agents (Continued)

Drug, Toxicity Notes	Percent Excreted Unchanged	Half-Life (Normal/ESRD)	Plasma Protein Binding	Volume of Distribution	Dose for Normal Renal Function	Method	Adjustment for Renal Failure GFR, mL/min >50	10-50	<10	Supplement for Dialysis
	%	h	%	L/kg						
Propofol	< 0.3	3-4.5/Unchanged	Unknown	3.0-14.4	2-2.5 mg/kg	D	100%	100%	100%	Hemo: Unknown CAPD: Unknown CAVH: Unknown
Pyridostigmine	80-90	1.5-2/6	Unknown	0.8-1.4	60-1500 mg/d	D	50%	35%	20%	Hemo: Unknown CAPD: Unknown CAVH: Unknown
Succinylcholine Renal excretion decreased by basic drugs. Hyperkalemia in ESRD.	None	3/Unknown	Unknown	Unknown	0.3-1.1 mg/kg load, then 0.04-0.07 mg/kg prn	D	100%	100%	100%	Hemo: Unknown CAPD: Unknown CAVH: Unknown
Sufentanil	1-2	1-2/Unchanged	92	1.7-5.2	1-30 μg/kg	D	100%	100%	100%	Hemo: Unknown CAPD: Unknown CAVH: Unknown
Tubocurarine Large or repetitive doses may result in prolonged effect. Recurarization may occur.	40-60	0.5-4/5.5	30-50	0.22-0.39	0.1-0.2 mg/kg	D	75%	50%	Avoid	Hemo: Unknown CAPD: Unknown CAVH: Unknown

For definitions of the abbreviations used in the tables, see page 14.

| Vecuronium | 25 | 0.5-1.3/Unchanged | 30 | 0.18-0.27 | 0.08-0.1 mg/kg load, then 0.01-0.05 mg/kg q12-15 min | D | 100% | 100% | 100% | Hemo: Unknown
CAPD: Unknown
CAVH: Unknown |

For definitions of the abbreviations used in the tables, see page 14.

Bibliography

Antimicrobial Agents

Antibacterial Antibiotics

Aminoglycoside Antibiotics

Amikacin

French MA, Cerra FB, Plaut ME, Schentag JJ. Amikacin and gentamicin accumulation pharmacokinetics and nephrotoxicity in critically ill patients. Antimicrob Agents Chemother. 1981;19:147-52.

Regeur L, Colding H, Jensen H, Kampmann JP. Pharmacokinetics of amikacin during hemodialysis and peritoneal dialysis. Antimicrob Agents Chemother. 1977;11:214-8.

Gentamicin

De Paepe M, Lameire N, Belpaire F, Bogaert M. Peritoneal pharmacokinetics of gentamicin in man. Clin Nephrol. 1983;19:107-9.

Pancorbo S, Comty C. Pharmacokinetics of gentamicin in patients undergoing continuous ambulatory peritoneal dialysis. Antimicrob Agents Chemother. 1981;19:605-7.

Thompson MI, Russo ME, Saxon BJ, Atkin-Thor E, Matsen JM. Gentamicin inactivation by piperacillin or carbenicillin in patients with end-stage renal disease. Antimicrob Agents Chemother. 1983;21:268-73.

Netilmicin

Luft FC, Brannon DR, Stropes LL, Costello RJ, Sloan RS, Maxwell DR. Pharmacokinetics of netilmicin in patients with renal impairment in patients on dialysis. Antimicrob Agents Chemother. 1978;14:403-7.

Tobramycin

Aarons L, Vozeh S, Wenk M, et al. Population pharmacokinetics of tobramycin. Br J Clin Pharmacokinet. 1989;28:305-14.

Brogden RN, Pender RM, Sawyer PR, Speight TM, Avery GS. Tobramycin: a review of its antibacterial and pharmakinetic properties and therapeutic use. Drugs. 1976;12:166-200.

Bunke CM, Aronoff GR, Brier ME, Sloan RS, Luft FC. Tobramycin kinetics during continuous ambulatory peritoneal dialysis. Clin Pharmacol Ther. 1983;34:110-6.

Cephalosporin Antibiotics

Cefaclor

Spyker DA, Gober LL, Scheld WM, Sande MA, Bolton WK. Pharmacokinetics of cefaclor in renal failure: effects of multiple doses and hemodialysis. Antimicrob Agents Chemother. 1982;21:278-81.

Cefadroxil

Cutler RE, Blair AD, Kelly MR. Cefadroxil kinetics in patients with renal insufficiency. Clin Pharmacol Ther. 1979;25(Suppl 1):514-21.

Leroy A, Humbert G, Godin M, Fillastre JP. Pharmacokinetics of cefadroxil in patients with impaired renal function. Antimicrob Chemother. 1982; 10(Suppl B):39-46.

Cefamandole

Czerwinski A, Federson J. Pharmacokinetics of cefamandole in patients with renal impairment. Antimicrob Agents Chemother. 1979;15:161-4.

Gambertoglio JG, Aziz NS, Lin ET, Grausz H, Naughton JL, Benet LZ. Cefamandole kinetics in uremic patients undergoing hemodialysis. Clin Pharmacol Ther. 1979;26:592-9.

Pancorbo S, Comty C. Pharmacokinetics of cefamandole in patients undergoing continuous ambulatory peritoneal dialysis. Perit Dialy Bull. 1983;3: 135-7.

Cefazolin

Brogard JM, Pinget M, Brandt C, Lavillaureix J. Pharmacokinetics of cefazolin in patients with renal failure: special reference to hemodialysis. J Clin Pharmacol. 1977;17:225-30.

Hiner LB, Baluarte HJ, Polinsky MS, Gruskin AB. Cefazolin in children with renal insufficiency. J Pediatr. 1980;96:335-9.

Kaye D, Wenger N, Agarwal B. Pharmacology of intraperitoneal cefazolin in patients undergoing peritoneal dialysis. Antimicrob Agents Chemother. 1978;14:318-21.

Cefepime

Barbhaiya RH, Knupp CA, Forgue ST, et al. Pharmacokinetics of cefepime in subjects with renal insufficiency. Clin Pharm Ther. 1990;48:268-76.

Barbhaiya RH, Forgue ST, Gleason CR, et al. Pharmacokinetics of cefepime after single and multiple intravenous administration in healthy subjects. Antimicrob Agents Chemother. 1992;36:552-7.

Barbhaiya RH, Knupp CA, Pfeffer M, et al. Pharmacokinetics of cefepime in patients undergoing continuous ambulatory peritoneal dialysis. Antimicrob Agents Chemother. 1992;36:1387-91.

Cefixime

Faulkner RD, Bohaychuk W, Lanc RA, et al. Pharmacokinetics of cefixime in the young and elderly. J Antimicrob Chemother. 1988;21:787-94.

Guay DR, Meatherall RC, Harding GK, Brown GR. Pharmacokinetics of cefixime (CL284,635FK027) in healthy subjects and patients with renal insufficiency. Antimicrob Agents Chemother. 1986;30:485-90.

Cefmenoxime

Konish K. Pharmacokinetics of cefmenoxime in patients with impaired renal function and in those undergoing hemodialysis. Antimicrob Agents Chemother. 1986;30:901-5.

Cefmetazole

Halstenson CE, Guay DR, Opsahl JA, et al. Disposition of cefmetazole in healthy volunteers and patients with impaired renal function. Antimicrob Agents Chemother. 1990;34:519-23.

Cefonicid

Barriere SL, Gambertoglio JG, Alexander DP, Stagg RJ, Conte JE Jr. Pharmacokinetic disposition of cefonicid in patients with renal failure and receiving hemodialysis. Rev Infect Dis. 1984;6(Suppl 4):S809-15.

Blair AD, Maxwell BM, Forland SC, Jacob L, Cutler RE. Cefonicid kinetics in subjects with normal and impaired renal function. Clin Pharmacol Ther. 1984;35:798-803.

Cefoperazone

Greenfield RA, Gerber AU, Craig WA. Pharmacokinetics of cefoperazone in patients with normal and impaired hepatic and renal function. Rev Infect Dis. 1983;5:S127-36.

Keller E, Jansen A, Pelz K, Hoppe-Seyler G, Schollmeyer P. Intraperitoneal and intravenous cefoperazone kinetics during continuous ambulatory peritoneal dialysis. Clin Pharmacol Ther. 1984;35:208-13.

Spyker DA, Richmond JD, Scheld WM, Bolton WK. Pharmacokinetics of multiple-dose cefoperazone in hemodialysis patients. Am J Nephrol. 1985;5:355-60.

Trollfors B, Ahlemen J, Alestig K. Renal function during cefoperazone treatment. J Antimicrob Chemother. 1982;9:485-7.

Ceforanide

Estey EH, Weaver SS, LeBlanc BM, Brown N, Ho DH, Bodey GP. Ceforanide kinetics. Clin Pharmacol Ther. 1981;30:398-403.

Hawkins SS, Alford RH, Stone WJ, Smyth RD, Pfeffer M. Ceforanide kinetics in renal insufficiency. Clin Pharmacol Ther. 1981;30:468-74.

Cefotaxime

Albin HC, Demotes-Mainard FM, Bouchet JL, Vincon GA, Martin-Dupont C. Pharmacokinetics of intravenous and intraperitoneal cefotaxime in chronic ambulatory peritoneal dialysis. Clin Pharmacol Ther. 1985;38: 285-9.

Doluisio JT. Clinical pharmacokinetics of cefotaxime in patients with normal and reduced renal function. Rev Infect Dis. 1982;4(Suppl):S33-45.

Ings RM, Fillastre JP, Godin M, Leroy A, Humbert G. The pharmacokinetics of cefotaxime and its metabolites in subjects with normal and impaired renal function. Rev Infect Dis. 1982;4(Suppl):S379-91.

Peterson J, Stewart RD, Catto GR, Edward N. Pharmacokinetics of intraperitoneal cefotaxime treatment of peritonitis in patients on continuous ambulatory peritoneal dialysis. Nephron. 1985;40:79-82.

Rodondi LC, Flaherty JF, Schoenfeld P, et al. Influence of coadministration on the pharmacokinetics of mezlocillin and cefotaxime in healthy volunteers and in patients with renal failure. Clin Pharmacol Ther. 1989;45: 527-34.

Cefotetan

Browning MJ, Hoh HA, White LD, et al. Pharmacokinetics of cefotetan in patients with end-stage renal failure on maintenance dialysis. J Antimicrob Chemother. 1986;18:103-6.

Ohkawa M, Hirano S, Tokunaga S, et al. Pharmacokinetics of cefotetan in normal subjects and patients with impaired renal function. Antimicrob Agents Chemother. 1983;23:31-5.

Ward A, Richards DM. Cefotetan: a review of its antimicrobial activity, pharmacokinetic properties and therapeutic uses. Drugs. 1985;30: 382-426.

Cefoxitin

Arvidsson A, Alvan G, Tranaeus A, Malmborg AS. Pharmacokinetic studies of cefoxitin in continuous ambulatory peritoneal dialysis. Eur J Clin Pharmacol. 1985;28:333-7.

Brogden RN, Heel RC, Speight TM, Avery GS. Cefoxitin: a review of its antibacterial activity, pharmacological properties and therapeutic use. Drugs. 1979;17:1-37.

Fillastre JP, Leroy A, Godin M, Oksenhendler G, Humbert G. Pharmacokinetics of cefoxitin sodium in normal subjects and in uraemic patients. J Antimicrob Chemother. 1978;4(Suppl B):79-83.

Cefpodoxime

Borin MT, Hughes GS, Kelloway JS, et al. Disposition of cefpodoxime proxetil in hemodialysis patients. J Clin Pharmacol. 1992;32:1038-44.

St. Peter JV, Borin MT, Hughes GS, et al. Disposition of cefpodoxime proxetil in healthy volunteers and patients with impaired renal function. Antimicrob Agents Chemother. 1992;36:126-31.

Cefprozil

Shyu WC, Pittmen KA, Wilber RB, et al. Pharmacokinetics of cefprozil in healthy subjects and patients with renal impairment. J Clin Pharmacol. 1991;31:362-71.

Ceftazidime

Ackerman BH, Ross J, Tofte RW, Rotschafer JC. Effect of decreased renal function on the pharmacokinetics of ceftazidime. Antimicrob Agents Chemother. 1984;25:785-6.

Lin MS, Wang LS, Huang JD. Single and multiple dose pharmacokinetics of ceftazidime in infected patients with varying degrees of renal function. J Clin Pharmacol. 1989;29:331-7.

Tourkantonis A, Nikolaidis P. Pharmacokinetics of ceftazidime in patients undergoing peritoneal dialysis. J Antimicrob Chemother. 1983;12(Suppl A):263-7.

Ceftizoxime

Gross ML, Somani P, Ribner BS, Raeader R, Freimer EH, Higgins JT Jr. Ceftizoxime elimination kinetics in continuous ambulatory peritoneal dialysis. Clin Pharmacol Ther. 1983;34:673-80.

Kowalsky SF, Echols RM, Venezia AR, Andrews EA. Pharmacokinetics of ceftizoxime in subjects with various degrees of renal function. Antimicrob Agents Chemother. 1983;24:151-5.

Ceftriaxone

Stoeckel K, Koup JR. Pharmacokinetics of ceftriaxone in patients with renal and liver insufficiency and correlations with a physiologic nonlinear protein binding model. Am J Med. 1984;77:26-32.

Ti TY, Fortin L, Kreeft JH, East DS, Ogilvie RI, Somerville PJ. Kinetics disposition of intravenous ceftriaxone in normal subjects and patients with renal failure on hemodialysis or peritoneal dialysis. Antimicrob Agents Chemother. 1984;25:83-7.

Cefuroxime

Chan MK, Browning AK, Poole CJ, Matheson LA, Li CS, Biallod RA. Cefuroxime pharmacokinetics in continuous and intermittent peritoneal dialysis. Nephron. 1985;41:161-5.

Walstad RA, Nilsen OG, Berg KJ. Pharmacokinetics and clinical effects of cefuroxime in patients with severe renal insufficiency. Eur J Clin Pharmacol. 1983;24:391-8.

Cephalexin

Bailey RR, Gower PE, Dash CH. The effects of impairment of renal function and haemodialysis on serum and urine levels of cephalexin. Postgrad Med J. 1970;46(Suppl):60-4.

Bunke CM, Aronoff GR, Brier ME, Sloan RS, Luft FC. Cefazolin and cephalexin kinetics in continuous ambulatory peritoneal dialysis. Clin Pharmacol Ther. 1983;33:66-72.

Drew PJ, Casewell MW, Desai N, Houang ET, Simpson CN, Marsh FP. Cephalexin for the oral treatment of CAPD peritonitis. J Antimicrob Chemother. 1984;13:153-9.

Cephalothin

Munch R, Steurer J, Luthy R, Siegenthaler W, Kuhlmann U. Serum and dialyzate concentrations of intraperitoneal cephalothin in patients undergoing continuous ambulatory peritoneal dialysis. Clin Nephrol. 1983;20:40-3.

Rankin LI, Swain RR, Luft FC. Effect of cephalothin on measurement of creatinine concentration. Antimicrob Agents Chemother. 1979;15:666-9.

Venuto RC, Plaut M. Cephalothin handling in patients undergoing hemodialysis. Antimicrob Agents Chemother. 1970;10:50-2.

Cephapirin

Bergan T, Orjavik O, Brodwall EK. Pharmacokinetics of cephapirin in patients with normal and impaired renal functions. Arzneimittelforschung. 1981;31:1773-6.

McCloskey RV, Terry EE, McCracken AW, Sweeney MJ, Forland MF. Effect of hemodialysis and renal failure on serum and urine concentrations of cephapirin sodium. Antimicrob Agents Chemother. 1972;1:90-3.

Cephradine

Johnson CA, Welling PG, Zimmerman SW. Pharmacokinetics of oral cephradine in continuous ambulatory peritoneal dialysis patients. Nephron. 1984;38:57-61.

Searle M, Raman GV. Oral treatment of peritonitis complicating continuous ambulatory peritoneal dialysis. Clin Nephrol. 1985;23:241-4.

Solomon AE, Briggs JD. The administration of cephradine to patients in renal failure. Br J Clin Pharmacol. 1975;2:443-8.

Moxalactam (Latamoxef)

Aronoff GR, Sloan RS, Luft FC. Pharmacokinetics of moxalactam in patients with normal and impaired renal function. J Infect Dis. 1981;145:365-9.

Aronoff GR, Sloan RS, Mong SA, Luft FC, Kleit SA. Moxalactam pharmacokinetics during hemodialysis. Antimicrob Agents Chemother. 1981;19:575-7.

Jones TE, Milne RW, Mudaliar Y, Sansom LN. Moxalactam kinetics during continuous ambulatory peritoneal dialysis after intraperitoneal administration. Antimicrob Agents Chemother. 1985;28:293-8.

Miscellaneous Antibacterial Antibiotics

Golper TA, Gleason JR, Vincent HH, Vos MC. Drug removal during high efficiency and high flux hemodialysis. Contemp Iss Nephrol. 1993;27:175-208.

St. Peter WL, Redic-Kill KA, Haltenson CE. Clinical pharmacokinetics of antibiotics in patients with impaired renal function. Clin Pharmacokinet. 1992;22:169-210.

Keane WF, Everett ED, Golper TA, et al. Peritoneal dialysis-related peritonitis treatment recommendations, 1993 update. Perit Dial Int. 1993;13:14-28.

Aztreonam

Brogden RN, Heel RC. Aztreonam: a review of its antibacterial activity, pharmacokinetic properties and therapeutic use. Drugs. 1986;31:96-130.

Fillastre JP, Leroy A, Baudoin C, et al. Pharmacokinetics of aztreonam in patients with chronic renal failure. Clin Pharmacokinet. 1985;10:91-100.

Gerig JS, Bolton ND, Swabb EA, Scheld WM, Bolton WK. Effect of hemodialysis and peritoneal dialysis on aztreonam pharmacokinetics. Kidney Int. 1984;26:308-18.

Azithromycin

Cooper MA, Nye K, Andrews JM, Wise R. The pharmacokinetics and inflammatory fluid penetration of orally administered azithromycin. J Antimicrob Chemother. 1990;26:533-8.

Foulds G, Shephard RM, Johnson RB. The pharmacokinetics of azithromycin in human serum and tissue. J Antimicrob Chemother. 1990;25(Suppl A):73-82.

Chloramphenicol

Ambrose PJ. Clinical pharmacokinetics of chloramphenicol and chloramphenicol succinate. Clin Pharmacokinet. 1984;9:222-38.

Grafnetterova J, Vodrazka Z, Jandova D, Shuck O, Tomasek R, Lachmanova J. The binding of chloramphenicol to serum proteins in patients with chronic renal insufficiency. Clin Nephrol. 1976;6:448-50.

Slaughter RL, Cerra FB, Koup JR. Effect of hemodialysis on total body clearance of chloramphenicol. Am J Hosp Pharm. 1980;37:1083-6.

Cinoxacin

Sisca TA, Heel RC, Romankiewicz JA. Cinoxacin: a review of its pharmacological properties and therapeutic efficacy in the treatment of urinary tract infections. Drugs. 1983;25:544-69.

Ciprofloxacin

Aronoff GR, Kenner CH, Sloan RS, Pottratz ST. Multiple-dose ciprofloxacin kinetics in normal subjects. Clin Pharmacol Ther. 1984;36:384-8.

Forrest A, Weir M, Plaisance KI, et al. Relationship between renal function and disposition of oral ciprofloxacin. Antimicrob Agents Chemother. 1988;32:1537-40.

Golper TA, Hartstein AI, Moorthland VH, Christensen JM. Effects of antacids and dialysate dwell times on multiple dose pharmacokinetics of oral ciprofloxacin in patients on CAPD. Antimicrob Agents Chemother. 1987;31:1787-90.

Hoffken G, Lode H, Prinzing C, Borner K, Koeppe P. Pharmacokinetics of ciprofloxacin after oral and parenteral administration. Antimicrob Agents Chemother. 1985;27:375-9.

Clarithromycin

Ferrero JL, Bopp BA, Marsh KC, et al. Metabolism and disposition of clarithromycin in man. Drug Metab Dispos Biol Fate Chem. 1990;18: 441-6.

Chu SY, Sennello LT, Bunnell ST, et al. Pharmacokinetics of clarithromycin, a new macrolide after single ascending oral doses. Antimicrob Agents Chemother. 1992;36:2447-53.

Clavulanic Acid

Dalet F, Amado E, Cabrera E, et al. Pharmacokinetics of the combination of ticarcillin with clavulanic acid in renal insufficiency. J Antimicrob Chemother. 1986;17(Suppl C):57-64.

Jackson D, Cooper DL, Filer CW, Langley PF. Augmentin, absorption, excretion and pharmacokinetic studies in man. Postgrad Med. 1984; 76(Suppl):51-70.

Slaughter RL, Kohli R, Brass C. Effects of hemodialysis on the pharmaco-kinetics of amoxicillin/clavulanic acid combination. Ther Drug Monit. 1984;6:424-7.

Clindamycin

Golper TA, Sewell DL, Fisher PB, Wolfson M. Incomplete activation of intraperitoneal clindamycin phosphate during peritoneal dialysis. Am J Nephrol. 1984;6:38-42.

Roberts A, Eastwood J, Gower P, Fenton C, Curtis J. Serum and plasma concentrations of clindamycin following a single intramuscular injection of clindamycin phosphate in maintenance hemodialysis patients and nor-mal subjects. Eur J Clin Pharmacol. 1978;14:435-9.

Erythromycin

Kanfer A, Stamatakis G, Torlotin JC, et al. Changes in erythromycin pharmacokinetics induced by renal failure. Clin Nephrol. 1987;27:147-50.

Krobath PD, McNeil MA, Kreeger A, Dominquez J, Rault R. Hearing loss and erythromycin pharmacokinetics in a patient receiving hemodialysis. Arch Intern Med. 1983;143:1263-5.

Welling PG, Craig WA. Pharmacokinetics of intravenous erythromycin. J Pharm Sci. 1978;17:1057-9.

Fleroxacin

Stuck AE, Frey FJ, Heizmann P, et al. Pharmacokinetics and metabolism of intravenous and oral fleroxacin in patients on continuous ambulatory peri-toneal dialysis. Antimicrob Agents Chemother. 1989;33:373-81.

Imipenem

Gibson TP, Demetriades JL, Bland JA. Imipenem/cilastin: pharmacokinetic profile in renal insufficiency. Am J Med. 1985;78:(Suppl 6A):54-61.

Verbist L, Verpooten GA, Giuliano RA, et al. Pharmacokinetics and tolerance after repeated doses of imipenem/cilastin in patients with severe renal failure. J Antimicrob Chemother. 1986;18:(Suppl E):115-20.

Lincomycin

Malacoff RF, Finkelstein FO, Andriole VT. Effect of peritoneal dialysis on serum levels of tobramycin and lincomycin. Antimicrob Agents Chemother. 1975;8:574-80.

Meropenum

Chimata M, Vagase M, Suzuki Y, et al. Pharmacokinetics of meropenum in patients with various degrees of renal function including patients with end stage renal disease. Antimicrob Agents Chemother. 1993;37:229-33.

Christensson BA, Nilsson-Ehle I, Hutchison M, et al. Pharmacokinetics of meropenum in subjects with various degrees of renal impairment. Antimicrob Agents Chemother. 1992;36:1532-37.

Methenamine Mandelate

Hamilton-Miller JM, Brumfitt W. Methenamine and its salts as urinary tract antiseptics: variables affecting the antibacterial activity of formaldehyde, mandelic acid, and hippuric acid in vitro. Invest Urol. 1977;14:287-91.

Metronidazole

Guay DR, Meatherall RC, Baxter H, Jacyk WR, Penner B. Pharmacokinetics of metronidazole in patients undergoing continuous ambulatory peritoneal dialysis. Antimicrob Agents Chemother. 1984;25:306-10.

Houghton GW, Dennis MJ, Gabriel P. Pharmacokinetics of metronidazole in patients with varying degrees of renal failure. Br J Clin Pharmacol. 1985;19:203-9.

Lau AH, Chang CW, Sabatini S. Hemodialysis clearance of metronidazole and its metabolites. Antimicrob Agents Chemother. 1986;29:235-8.

Nalidixic Acid

Dash H, Mills J. Severe metabolic acidosis associated with nalidixic acid overdose [Letter]. Ann Intern Med. 1976;84:570-1.

Ferry N, Cuisinaud G, Pozet N, Zech PY, Sassard J. Nalidixic acid kinetics after single and repeated oral doses. Clin Pharmacol Ther. 1981;29:695-8.

Nitrofurantoin

Conklin JD. The pharmacokinetics of nitrofurantoin and its related bioavailability. Antibiot Chemother. 1978;25:233-52.

Liedtke RK, Ebel S, Missler B, Haase W, Stein L. Single-dose pharmacokinetics of macrocrystalline nitrofurantoin formulations. Arzneimittelforschung. 1980;20:833-6.

Toole JF, Parrish ML. Nitrofurantoin polyneuropathy. Neurology. 1973;23: 554-9.

Norfloxacin

Holmes B, Brogden RN, Richards DM. Norfloxacin: a review of its antibacterial activity, pharmacokinetic properties and therapeutic use. Drugs. 1985;30:482-513.

Ofloxacin

Fillastre JP, Leroy A, Hambert G. Ofloxacin pharmacokinetics in renal failure. Antimicrob Agents Chemother. 1987;31:156-60.

Lameire N, Rosenkranz B, Malercyk V, et al. Ofloxacin pharmacokinetics in chronic renal failure and dialysis. Clin Pharmacokinet. 1991;21:357-71.

Lode H, Hoffken G, Prinzing C, et al. Comparative pharmacokinetics of new quinolones. Drugs. 1987;34(Suppl 1):21-5.

White LD, MacGowan AP, Macket IG, Reeves DS. The pharmacokinetics of ofloxacin, desmethyl ofloxacin and ofloxacin N-oxide in haemodialysis patients with end-state renal failure. J Antimicrob Chemother. 1988; 22(Suppl C):65-72.

Spectinomycin

Kusumi R, Metzler C, Fass R. Pharmacokinetics of spectinomycin in volunteers with renal insufficiency. Chemotherapy. 1981;27:95-8.

Sulbactam

Reitberg DP, Marble DA, Schultz RW, et al. Pharmacokinetics of cefoperazone (2.0 g) and sulbactam (1.0 g) coadministered to subjects with normal renal function, patients with decreased renal function, and patients with end-stage renal disease on hemodialysis. Antimicrob Agents Chemother. 1988;32:503-9.

Wright N, Wise R. Elimination of sulbactam alone and combined with ampicillin in patients with renal dysfunction. J Antimicrob Chemother. 1983; 11:583-7.

Sulfonamides and Trimethoprim-Sulfamethoxazole

Berglund F, Killander J, Pompeius R. Effect of trimethoprim-sulfamethoxazole on renal excretion of creatinine in man. J Urol. 1975;114:802-8.

Halstenson CE, Blevins RB, Salem NG, Matzke GR. Trimethoprim-sulfamethoxazole pharmacokinetics during continuous ambulatory peritoneal dialysis. Clin Nephrol. 1984;22:239-43.

Siber GR, Gorham CC, Ericson JF, Smith AL. Pharmacokinetics of intravenous trimethoprim-sulfamethoxazole in children and adults with normal and impaired renal function. Rev Infect Dis. 1982;4:566-78.

Tazobactam

Johnson CA, Haltenson CE, Kelloway BE, et al. Single dose pharmacokinetics of piperacillin and tazobactam in patients with renal disease. Clin Pharmacol Ther. 1992;51:32-41.

Sorgel F, Kinzig M. The chemistry, pharmacokinetics and tissue distribution of piperacillin/tazobactam. J Antimicrob Chemother. 1993;31(Suppl A):39-60.

Teicoplanin

Bonati M, Traina GL, Gentile MG, et al. Pharmacokinetics of intraperitoneal teicoplanin in patients with chronic renal failure on continuous ambulatory peritoneal dialysis. Br J Pharmacol. 1988;25:761-5.

Domart Y, Pierre C, Clair B, et al. Pharmacokinetics of teicoplanin in critically ill patients with varying degrees of renal impairment. Antimicrob Agents Chemother. 1987;31:1600-4.

Falcoz C, Ferry N, Pozet N, et al. Pharmacokinetics of teicoplanin in renal failure. Antimicrob Agents Chemother. 1987;31:1255-62.

McNulty CA, Garden GM, Wise R, et al. The pharmacokinetics and tissue penetration of teicoplanin. J Antimicrob Chemother. 1985;16:743-9.

Trimethoprim

Myre SA, McCann J, First MR, Cluxton RJ. Effect of trimethoprim on serum creatinine in healthy and chronic renal failure volunteers. Ther Drug Monit. 1987;9:161-5.

Vancomycin

Brown DL, Manro LS. Vancomycin dosing chart for use in patients with renal impairment. Am J Kidney Dis. 1988;11:15-9.

Cutler NR, Narang PK, Lesko LJ, Ninos M, Power M. Vancomycin disposition: the importance of age. Clin Pharmacol Ther. 1984;36:803-10.

Golper TA, Noonan HM, Elzinga L, et al. Vancomycin pharmacokinetics: renal handling and nonrenal clearances in normal human subjects. Clin Pharmacol Ther. 1988;43:565-70.

Magera BE, Arroyo JC, Rosansky SJ, Postic B. Vancomycin pharmacokinetics in patients with peritonitis on peritoneal dialysis. Antimicrob Agents Chemother. 1983;23:710-4.

Moellering RC Jr, Krogstad DJ, Greenblatt DJ. Vancomycin therapy in patients with impaired renal function: a nomogram for dosage. Ann Intern Med. 1981;94:343-6.

Penicillins

Amoxicillin, Ampicillin, and Amoxicillin/Clavula

Davies BE, Boon R, Horton R, et al. Pharmacokinetics of amoxicillin and clavulanic acid in haemodialysis patients following intravenous administration of Augmentin. Br J Clin Pharmacol. 1988;26:385-90.

Francke E, Appel GB, Neu HC. Kinetics of intravenous amoxicillin in patients on long-term dialysis. Clin Pharmacol Ther. 1979;26:31-5.

Humbert G, Spyker DA, Fillastre JP, Leroy A. Pharmacokinetics of amoxicillin: dosage nomogram for patients with impaired renal function. Antimicrob Agents Chemother. 1979;15:28-33.

Azlocillin

Leroy A, Humbert G, Godin M, Fillastre JP. Pharmacokinetics of azlocillin in subjects with normal and impaired renal function. Antimicrob Agents Chemother. 1980;17:344-9.

Whelton A, Stout RL, Delgado FA. Azlocillin kinetics during extracorporeal hemodialysis and peritoneal dialysis. J Antimicrob Chemother. 1983; 11(Suppl B):89-95.

Mezlocillin

Aronoff GR, Sloan RS, Stanish RA, Fineberg NS. Mezlocillin dose dependent elimination kinetics in renal impairment. Eur J Clin Pharmacol. 1982; 21:505-9.

Kampf D, Schurig R, Weihermuller K, Forester D. Effects of impaired renal function, hemodialysis, and peritoneal dialysis on the pharmacokinetics of mezlocillin. Antimicrob Agents Chemother. 1980;18:81-7.

Nafcillin

Rudnick M, Morrison G, Walker B, Singer I. Renal failure hemodialysis and nafcillin kinetics. Clin Pharmacol Ther. 1976;20:413-23.

Piperacillin

Aronoff GR, Sloan RS, Brier ME, Luft FC. The effect of piperacillin dose on elimination kinetics in renal impairment. Eur J Clin Pharmacol. 1983;24:543-7.

Francke EL, Appel GB, Neu HC. Pharmacokinetics of intravenous piperacillin patients undergoing chronic hemodialysis. Antimicrob Agents Chemother. 1979;16:788-91.

Ticarcillin

English J, Gilbert DN, Kohlhepp J, et al. Attenuation of experimental tobramycin nephrotoxicity by ticarcillin. Antimicrob Agents Chemother. 1985; 27:897-902.

Parry MF, Neu HC. Pharmacokinetics of ticarcillin in patients with abnormal renal function. J Infect Dis. 1976;133:46-9.

Quinolone Antibiotics

Eliopoulos GM. New quinolones: pharmacology, pharmacokinetics and dosing in patients with renal insufficiency. Rev Infect Dis. 1988;10(Suppl 1): S102-5.

Wolfson JS, Hooper DC. Pharmacokinetics of quinolones: newer aspects. Eur J Clin Microbiol Infect Dis. 1991;10:267-74.

Lomefloxacin

Blum RA, Schultz RW, Schentag JJ. Pharmacokinetics of lomefloxacin in renally compromised patients. Antimicrob Agents Chemother. 1990;34: 2364-8.

Pefloxacin

Montay G, Jacquot C, Bariety J, Cunci R. Pharmacokinetics of pefloxacin in renal insufficiency. Eur J Clin Pharmacol. 1985;29:345-9.

Schmit JL, Hary L, Bou P, et al. Pharmacokinetics of single dose intravenous, oral and intraperitoneal pefloxacin in patients on chronic ambulatory peritoneal dialysis. Antimicrob Agents Chemother. 1991;35:1492-4.

Antifungal Antibiotics

Terrell CL, Hughes CE. Antifungal agents used for deep seated mycotic infections. Mayo Clin Proc. 1992;67:69-91.

Amphotericin

Block ER, Bennett JE, Livoti LG, Klein WJ, MacGregor RR, Henderson L. Flucytosine and amphotericin B: hemodialysis effects on the plasma concentration and clearance: studies in man. Ann Intern Med. 1974;80:613-7.

Morgan DJ, Ching MS, Raymond K, et al. Elimination of amphotericin B in impaired renal function. Clin Pharmacol Ther. 1983;34:248-53.

Muther RS, Bennett WM. Peritoneal clearance of amphotericin B and 5-fluorocytosine. West J Med. 1980;133:157-60.

Fluconazole

Humphrey MJ, Jerons S, Tarbit MH. Pharmacokinetic evaluation of UK-49, 858, a metabolically stable triazole antifungal drug, in animals and humans. Antimicrob Agents Chemother. 1985;28:648-53.

Thomas MG, Ellis-Pegler RB. Fluconazole treatment of *Candida glabrata* peritonitis. J Antimicrob Chemother. 1989;24:94-5.

Flucytosine

Cutler RE, Blair AD, Kelly MR. Flucytosine kinetics in subjects with normal and impaired renal function. Clin Pharmacol Ther. 1978;24:333-42.

Itraconazole

Boelaert J, Schurgers M, Matthys E, et al. Itraconazole pharmacokinetics in patients with renal dysfunction. Antimicrob Agents Chemother. 1988;32:1595-7.

Hardin TC, Graybill JR, Fetchick R, et al. Pharmacokinetics of itraconazole following oral administration to normal volunteers. Antimicrob Agents Chemother. 1988;32:1310-3.

Heykants J, Van Peer A, Van de Vilde V, et al. Clinical pharmacokinetics of itranconazole: a review. Mycoses. 1989;32(Suppl 1):67-87.

Ketoconazole

Daneshmend TK, Warnock DW, Turner A, Roberts CJ. Pharmacokinetics of ketoconazole in normal subjects. J Antimicrob Chemother. 1981;8:299-304.

Heel RC, Brogden RN, Carmine A, Morley PA, Speight TM, Avery GS. Ketoconazole: a review of its therapeutic efficacy in superficial and systemic fungal infections. Drugs. 1982;23:1-36.

Johnson RJ, Blair AD, Ahmad S. Ketoconazole kinetics in chronic peritoneal dialysis. Clin Pharmacol Ther. 1985;37:325-9.

Miconazole

Lewis PJ, Boelaert J, Daneels R. Pharmacokinetic profile of intravenous miconazole in man: comparison of normal subjects and patients with renal insufficiency. Eur J Clin Pharmacol. 1976;10:49-54.

Antiparasitic Antibiotics

Pentamidine

Conte JE, Upton RA, Lin ET. Pentamidine pharmacokinetics in patients with AIDS with impaired renal function. J Infect Dis. 1987;156:890-5.

Antituberculous Antibiotics

Ethambutol

Lee CS, Marbury TC, Benet LZ. Clearance calculations in hemodialysis: application to blood, plasma, and dialysate measurements for ethambutol. J Pharmacokinet Biopharm. 1980;8:69-81.

Isoniazid

Gold CH, Buchanan N, Tringham V, Viljoen M, Struckwold B, Moodley GP. Isoniazid pharmacokinetics in patients with chronic renal failure. Clin Nephrol. 1976;6:365-9.

Rifampin

Acocella G. Clinical pharmacokinetics of rifampicin. Clin Pharmacokinet. 1978;3:108-27.

Antiviral Antibiotics

Acyclovir

Kransny HC, Liao S, Demiranda P, Laskin OL, Whelton A, Lietman PS. Influence of hemodialysis on acyclovir pharmacokinetics in patients with chronic renal failure. Am J Med. 1982;73:202-4.

Laskin OL. Clinical pharmacokinetics of acyclovir. Clin Pharmacokinet. 1983;8:187-201.

Amantadine

Horadam VW, Sharp JG, Smilack JD, McAnalley BH, Garriott JC, Stephens MK. Pharmacokinetics of amantadine hydrochloride in subjects with normal and impaired renal function. Ann Intern Med. 1981;94:454-8.

Wu MJ, Ing TS, Soung LS, Daugirdas JT, Hano JE, Gandhi VC. Amantadine hydrochloride pharmacokinetics in patients with impaired renal function. Clin Nephrol. 1982;17:19-23.

Didanosine

Hartman NR, Yarchoan R, Pluda JM, et al. Pharmacokinetics of 2',3'-dideoxyadenosine and 2'-3'-dideoxyinosine in patients with severe human immunodeficiency virus infection. Clin Pharmacol Ther. 1990;47:647-54.

Foscarnet

Ringden O, Lonnquist B, Paulin T, et al. Pharmacokinetic, safety and preliminary clinical experiences using foscarnet in the treatment of cytomegalovirus infections in bone marrow and renal transplant recipients. J Antimicrob Chemother. 1986;17:373-87.

Jacobson MA, Crowe S, Levy J, et al. Effect of foscarnet therapy on infection with human immunodeficiency virus in patients with AIDS. J Infect Dis. 1988;158:862-5.

Palestine AG, Polis MA, De Smet MD, et al. A randomized, controlled trial of foscarnet in treatment of cytomegalovirus retinitis in patients with AIDS. Ann Intern Med. 1991;115:665-73.

Ganciclovir

Fletcher C, Sawchuk R, Chinnock MT, et al. Human pharmacokinetics of the antiviral drug DHPG. Clin Pharmacol Ther. 1986;40:281-6.

Jackson MA, DeMiranda P, Cederberg DM, et al. Human pharmacokinetics and tolerance of oral ganciclovir. Antimicrob Agents Chemother. 1987; 31:1251-4.

Lake KD, Fletcher CV, Love KR, et al. Ganciclovir pharmacokinetics during renal impairment. Antimicrob Agents Chemother. 1988;32:1899-900.

Ribavirin

Kramer TH, Gaar GG, Ray CG, et al. Hemodialysis clearance of intravenously administered ribavirin. Antimicrob Agents Chemother. 1990;34: 489-90.

Laskin OL, Longstreth JA, Hart CC, et al. Ribavirin disposition in high risk patients for acquired immunodeficiency syndrome. Clin Pharmacol Ther. 1987;41:546-55.

Lertora JJ, Rege AB, La Cour JT, et al. Pharmacokinetics and long term tolerance to ribavirin in asymptomatic patients infected with immunodeficiency virus. Clin Pharmacol Ther. 1991;50:442-9.

Paroni R, Del Puppo M, Borght C, et al. Pharmacokinetics of ribavirin and urinary excretion of the major metabolite 1,2,4-triazole-3-carboxamide in normal volunteers. Int J Clin Pharmacol Ther Toxicol. 1989;27:302-7.

Roberts RB, Laskin OL, Laurence J, et al. Ribavirin pharmacodynamics in high risk patients for acquired immunodeficiency syndrome. Clin Pharmacol Ther. 1987;42:365-73.

Vidarabine

Aronoff GR, Szwed JJ, Nelson RL, Marcus EL, Kleit SA. Hypoxanthine-arabinoside pharmacokinetics after adenine arabinoside administration to a patient with renal failure. Antimicrob Agents Chemother. 1980;18:212-4.

Zidovudine

Gallicano KD, Tobe S, Saha J, et al. Pharmacokinetics of single and chronic dose zidovudine in two HIV+ patients undergoing CAPD. J Acquir Immune Defic Syndr. 1992;5:242-50.

Gleason J, Brier ME. Zidovudine: therapeutic recommendations for its use in renal failure. Semin Dialysis. 1990;3:101-4.

Klecker RW, Collins JM, Vorchoan R, et al. Plasma and CSF pharmacokinetics of 3-azido-3-deoxy-thymidine: a novel pyrimidine analog with potential application for treatment of patients with AIDS and related diseases. Clin Pharmacol Ther. 1987;41:407-12.

Kremer D, Munar MY, Kohlhepp SJ, et al. Zidovudine pharmacokinetics in five HIV seronegative patients undergoing continuous ambulatory peritoneal dialysis. Pharmacotherapy. 1992;12:56-60.

Singlas E, Pioger JC, Taburet AM, et al. Zidovudine disposition in patients with severe renal impairment: influence of hemodialysis. Clin Pharmacol Ther. 1989;46:190-7.

Antihypertensive and Cardiovascular Agents

Antihypertensive Drugs

Adrenergic and Serotoninergic Modulators

Clonidine

Langley MS, Heel RC. Transdermal clonidine: a preliminary review of its pharmacodynamic properties and therapeutic efficacy. Drugs. 1988;35:123-42.

Lowenthal DT, Matzek KM, MacGregor TR. Clinical pharmacokinetics of clonidine. Clin Pharmacokinet. 1988;14:287-310.

Doxazosin

Carlson RV, Bailey RR, Begg EJ, Cowlishaw MG, Sharman JR. Pharmacokinetics and effect on blood pressure of doxazosin in normal subjects and patients with renal failure. Clin Pharmacol Ther. 1986;40:561-6.

Oliver RM, Upward JW, Dewhurst AG, Honeywell R, Renwick AG, Waller DG. The pharmacokinetics of doxazosin in patients with hypertension and renal impairment. Br J Clin Pharm. 1990;29:417-22.

Young RA, Brogden RN. Doxazosin: a review of its pharmacodynamic and pharmacokinetic properties, and therapeutic efficacy in mild or moderate hypertension. Drugs. 1988;35:525-41.

Guanabenz

Holmes B, Brogden RN, Heel RC, Speight TM, Avery GS. Guanabenz: a review of its pharmacodynamic properties and therapeutic efficacy in hypertension. Drugs. 1983;26:212-29.

Guanadrel

Finnerty FA, Brogden RN. Guanadrel: a review of its pharmacodynamics and pharmacokinetic properties and therapeutic use in hypertension. Drugs. 1985;30:22-31.

Halstenson CE, Opsahl JA, Abraham PA, et al. Disposition of guanadrel in subjects with normal and impaired renal function. J Clin Pharmacol. 1989; 29:128-32.

Guanfacine

Carchman SH, Sica DA, Davis J, et al. Steady-state plasma levels and pharmacokinetics of guanfacine in patients with renal insufficiency. Nephron. 1989;53:18-23.

Sorkin EM, Heel RC. Guanfacine: a review of its pharmacodynamic and pharmacokinetic properties, and therapeutic efficacy in the treatment of hypertension. Drugs. 1986;31:301-36.

Ketanserin

Persson B, Heykants J, Hedner T. Clinical pharmacokinetics of ketanserin. Clin Pharmacokinet. 1991;20:263-79.

Ebihara A, Fugimura A. Metabolites of antihypertensive drugs. Clin Pharmacokinet. 1991;21:331-43.

Methyldopa

Myhre E, Rugstad HE, Hansen T. Clinical pharmacokinetics of methyldopa. Clin Pharmacokinet. 1982;7:221-33.

Prazosin

Lameire N, Gordts J. A pharmacokinetic study of prazosin in patients with varying degrees of chronic renal failure. Eur J Clin Pharmacol. 1986;31: 333-7.

Vincent J, Meredith PA, Reid JL, Elliot HL, Rubin PC. Clinical pharmacokinetics of prazosin. Clin Pharmacokinet. 1985;10:144-54.

Reserpine

Zsoter TT, Johnson GE, Deveber GA, Paul H. Excretion and metabolism of reserpine in renal failure. Clin Pharmacol Ther. 1973;14:325-30.

Terazosin

Achari R, Laddu A. Terazosin: a new alpha adrenoreceptor blocking drug. J Clin Pharmacol. 1992;32:520-3.

Titmarsh S, Monk JP. Terazosin: a review of its pharmacodynamic and pharmacokinetic properties, and therapeutic efficacy in essential hypertension. Drugs. 1987;33:461-77.

Angiotensin-Converting–Enzyme Inhibitors

Benazepril

Balfour JA, Goa KL. Benazepril: a review of its pharmacodynamic and pharmacokinetic properties and therapeutic efficacy in hypertension and congestive heart failure. Drugs. 1991;42:511-39.

Captopril

Brogden RN, Todd PA, Sorkin EM. Captopril: an update of its pharmacodynamic and pharmacokinetic properties, and therapeutic use in hypertension and congestive heart failure. Drugs. 1988;36:540-600.

Duchin KL, Pierides AM, Heald A, Signhvi SM, Rommel AJ. Elimination kinetics of captopril in patients with renal failure. Kidney Int. 1984;25:942-7.

Fujimura A, Kajiyama H, Ebihara A, Iwashita K, Nomura Y, Kawahara Y. Pharmacokinetics and pharmacodynamics of captopril in patients undergoing continuous ambulatory peritoneal dialysis. Nephron. 1986;44:324-8.

Enalapril

Fruncillo RJ, Rocci ML, Vlasses PH, et al. Disposition of enalapril and enalaprilat in renal insufficiency. Kidney Int. 1987;31:S117-22.

Mujais S, Quintanilla A, Zahid M, Koch K, Shaw W, Gibson T. Renal handling of enalaprilat. Am J Kidney Dis. 1992;19:121-5.

Todd PA, Goa KL. Enalapril: a reappraisal of its pharmacology and therapeutic use in hypertension. Drugs. 1992;43:346-61.

Fosinopril

Gehr T, Sica D, Grasela D, Fakhry I, Davis J, Duchin K. Fosinopril pharmacokinetics and pharmacodynamics in chronic ambulatory peritoneal dialysis patients. Eur J Clin Pharmacol. 1991;41:165-9.

Murdoch D, Mctavish D. Fosinopril. A review of its pharmacodynamic and pharmacokinetic properties and therapeutic potential in essential hypertension. Drugs. 1992;43:123-40.

Lisinopril

Chase SL, Sutton JD. Lisinopril: a new angiotensin-converting enzyme inhibitor. Pharmacotherapy. 1989;9:120-30.

Lancaster SG, Todd PA. Lisinopril: a preliminary review of its pharmacodynamic and pharmacokinetic properties, and therapeutic use in hypertension and congestive heart failure. Drugs. 1988;35:646-9.

Quinapril

Halstenson CE, Opsahl JA, Rachael K, et al. The pharmacokinetics of quinapril and its active metabolite quinaprilat in patients with varying degrees of renal function. J Clin Pharmacol. 1992;32:344-50.

Wadworth A, Brogden RN. Quinapril. A review of its pharmacological properties and therapeutic efficacy in cardiovascular disorders. Drugs. 1991;41:378-99.

Ramipril

Schunkert H, Kindler J, Gassmann M, et al. Pharmacokinetics of ramipril in hypertensive patients with renal insufficiency. Eur J Clin Pharmacol. 1989;37:249-56.

Todd PA, Benfield P. Ramipril: a review of its pharmacological properties and therapeutic efficacy in cardiovascular disorders. Drugs. 1990;39:110-35.

Beta Blockers

Acebutolol

Singh BN, Thoden WR, Ward A. Acebutolol: a review of its pharmocological properties and therapeutic efficacy in hypertension, angina pectoris and arrhythmia. Drugs. 1985;29:531-69.

Atenolol

Wadworth AN, Murdoch D, Brogden RN. Atenolol: a reappraisal of its pharmacological properties and therapeutic use in cardiovascular disorders. Drugs. 1991;41:468-510.

Bopindolol

Harron D, Goa KL, Langtry H. Bopindolol: a review of its pharmacodynamic and pharmacokinetic properties and therapeutic efficacy. Drugs. 1991; 41:130-49.

Carteolol

Hasenfub G, Schafer-Korting M, Knauf H, Mutschler E, Just H. Pharmacokinetics of carteolol in relation to renal function. Eur J Clin Pharmacol. 1985;29:461-5.

Celiprolol

Milne RJ, Buckley M. Celiprolol: an updated review of its pharmacodynamic and pharmacokinetic properties, and therapeutic efficacy in cardiovascular disease. Drugs. 1991;41:941-69.

Dilevalol

Chrisp P, Goa KL. Dilevalol: a review of its pharmacodynamic and pharmacokinetic properties and therapeutic potential in hypertension. Drugs. 1990;39:234-63.

Esmolol

Benfield P, Sorkin EM. Esmolol: a preliminary review of its pharmacodynamic and pharmacokinetic properties, and therapeutic efficacy. Drugs. 1987; 33:392-412.

Flaherty JF, Wong B, La Follette G, Warnock DG, Hulse JD, Gambertoglio JG. Pharmacokinetics of esmolol and ASL-8123 in renal failure. Clin Pharmacol Ther. 1989;45:321-7.

Labetalol

Goa KL, Benfield P, Sorkin EM. Labetalol: a reappraisal of its pharmacology, pharmacokinetics and therapeutic use in hypertension and ischaemic heart disease. Drugs. 1989;37:538-627.

Halstenson CE, Opsahl JA, Pence TV, et al. The disposition and dynamics of labetalol in patients on dialysis. Clin Pharmacol Ther. 1986;40:462-8.

Metoprolol

Regardh CG, Johnsson G. Clinical pharmacokinetics of metoprolol. Clin Pharmacokinet. 1980;5:557-69.

Nadolol

Frishman WH. Nadolol: a new B-adrenoceptor antagonist. N Engl J Med. 1981;305:678-82.

Penbutolol

Bernard N, Cuisinaud G, Pozet N, Zech PY, Sassard J. Pharmacokinetics of penbutolol and its metabolites in renal insufficiency. Eur J Clin Pharmacol. 1985;29:215-9.

Sclanz KD, Thomas RL. Penbutolol: a new beta-adrenergic blocking agent. DICP Ann Pharmacotherapy. 1990;24:403-8.

Pindolol

Ohnhaus EE, Heidemann H, Meier J, Maurer G. Metabolism of pindolol in patients with renal failure. Eur J Clin Pharmacol. 1982;22:423-8.

Propranolol

Stone WJ, Walle T. Massive propranolol metabolite retention during maintenance hemodialysis. Clin Pharmacol Ther. 1980;28:449-55.

Wood AJ, Vestal RE, Spannuth CL, Stone WJ, Wilkinson GR, Shand DG. Propranolol disposition in renal failure. Br J Clin Pharmacol. 1980;10: 561-6.

Sotalol

Singh BN, Deedwania P, Koonlawee N, Ward A, Sorkin EM. Sotalol: a review of its pharmacodynamic and pharmacokinetic properties, and therapeutic use. Drugs. 1987;34:311-49.

Vasodilators

Diazoxide

Pearson RM. Pharmacokinetics and response to diazoxide in renal failure. Clin Pharmacokinet. 1977;2:198-204.

Hydralazine

Ludden TM, McNay JL Jr, Shephard AM, Lin MS. Clinical pharmacokinetics of hydralazine. Clin Pharmacokinet. 1982;7:185-205.

Reece PA. Hydralazine and related compounds: chemistry, metabolism, and mode of action. Med Res Rev. 1981;1:73-96.

Minoxidil

Campese VM. Minoxidil: a review of its pharmacological properties and therapeutic use. Drugs. 1981;22:257-78.

Nitroprusside

Rindone JP, Sloane EP. Cyanide toxicity from sodium nitroprusside: risks and management. Ann Pharmacotherapy. 199;26:515-20.

Schulz V. Clinical pharmacokinetics of nitroprusside, cyanide, thiosulphate and thiocyanate. Clin Pharmacokinet. 1984;9:239-51.

Cardiovascular Drugs

Antiarrhythmic Agents

Bauman JL, Schoen MD, Hoon TJ. Practical optimization of antiarrhythmic drug therapy using pharmacokinetic principles. Clin Pharmacokinet. 1991; 20:151-66.

Amiodarone

Gill J, Heel RC, Fitton A. Amiodarone: an overview of its pharmacological properties and review of its therapeutic use in cardiac arrhythmias. Drugs. 1992;43:69-110.

Lesko LJ. Pharmacokinetic drug interactions with amiodarone. Clin Pharmacokinet. 1989;17:130-40.

Nattel S, Talajic M. Recent advances in understanding the pharmacology of amiodarone. Drugs. 1988;36:121-31.

Bretylium

Adir J, Narang PK, Josselson J. Nomogram for bretylium dosing in renal impairment. Ther Drug Monit. 1985;7:265-8.

Josselson J, Narang PK, Adir J, Yacobi A, Sadler JH. Bretylium kinetics in renal insufficiency. Clin Pharmacol Ther. 1983;33:144-50.

Rapeport WG. Clinical pharmacokinetics of bretylium. Clin Pharmacokinet. 1985;10:248-56.

Cibenzoline

Aronoff G, Brier M, Mayer ML, et al. Bioavailability and kinetics of cibenzoline in patients with normal and impaired renal function. J Clin Pharmacol. 1991; 31:38-44.

Harron DW, Brogden RN, Faulds D, Fitton A. Cibenzoline: a review of its pharmacological properties and therapeutic potential in arrhythmias. Drugs. 1992;43:734-759.

Massarella JW, Khoo KC, Aogaichi K, et al. Effect of renal impairment on the pharmacokinetics of cibenzoline. Clin Pharmacol Ther. 1988;43:317-23.

Disopyramide

Brogden RN, Todd PA. Disopyramide: a reappraisal of its pharmacodynamic and pharmacokinetic properties, and therapeutic use in cardiac arrhythmias. Drugs. 1987;34:151-87.

Siddoway LA, Woosley RL. Clinical pharmacokinetics of disopyramide. Clin Pharmacokinet. 1986;11:214-22.

Encainide

Brogden RN, Todd PA. Encainide: a review of its pharmacological properties and therapeutic efficacy. Drugs. 1987;34:519-38.

Roden DM, Woosley RL. Clinical pharmacokinetics of encainide. Clin Pharmacokinet. 1988;14:141-7.

Tartini A, Kesselbrenner M. Encainide-induced encephalopathy in a patient with chronic renal failure. Am J Kidney Dis. 1990;15:178-9.

Flecainide

Forland SC, Burgess E, Blair AD, et al. Oral flecainide pharmacokinetics in patients with impaired renal function. J Clin Pharmacol. 1988;28:259-67.

William AJ, McQuinn RL, Walls J. Pharmacokinetics of flecainide acetate in patients with severe renal impairment. Clin Pharmacol Ther. 1988;43:449-55.

Lidocaine

Bennett PN, Aarons LJ, Bending MR, Steiner JA, Rowland M. Pharmacokinetics of lidocaine and its deethylated metabolite: dose and time dependency studies in man. J Pharmacokinet Biopharm. 1982;10:265-81.

Lorcainide

Eriksson CD, Brogden RN. Lorcainide: a preliminary review of its pharmaco-dynamic properties and therapeutic efficacy. Drugs. 1984;72:279-300.

Mexiletine

Campbell RW. Mexiletine. N Engl J Med. 1987;316:29-34.

Evers J, Messer W, Aboudan F, Finke K. Mexiletin beiterminaler nierenin-suffizienz und verschiedenen dialysererfahren. Klin Wochenschr. 1989;67: 995-8.

Wang T, Wuellner D, Woosley RL, Stone WJ. Pharmacokinetics and non-dialyzability of mexiletine in renal failure. Clin Pharmacol Ther. 1985;37: 649-53.

Moricizine

Pieniaszek HJ Jr, McEntegart CM, Mayersohn M, Michael UF. Moricizine pharmacokinetics in renal insufficiency: reevaluation of elimination half-life. J Clin Pharmacol. 1992;32:412-4.

N-Acetyl Procainamide

Connolly SJ, Kates RE. Clinical pharmacokinetics of N-acetylprocainamide. Clin Pharmacokinet. 1982;7:205-20.

Domoto DT, Brown WW, Bruggensmith P. Removal of toxic levels of N-acetylprocainamide with continuous arteriovenous hemodiafiltration. Ann Intern Med. 1987;106:550-2.

Vlasses PH, Ferguson RK, Rocci ML Jr, Raja RM, Porter RS, Greenspan AM. Lethal accumulation of procainamide metabolite in severe renal insufficiency. Am J Nephrol. 1986;6:112-6.

Procainamide

Bauer LA, Black D, Gensler A, Sprinkle J. Influence of age, renal function and heart failure on procainamide clearance and N-acetylprocainamide serum concentrations. Int J Clin Pharmacol Ther Toxicol. 1989;27:213-6.

Raehl CL, Moorthy AV, Beirne GJ. Procainamide pharmacokinetics in patients on continuous ambulatory peritoneal dialysis. Nephron. 1986;44: 191-4.

Propafenone

Funck-Brentano C, Kroemer HK, Lee JT, Roden DM. Propafenone. N Engl J Med. 1990;322:518-25.

Hii J, Duff HJ, Burgess E. Clinical pharmacokinetics of propafenone. Clin Pharmacokinet. 1991;21:1-10.

Parker RB, McCollam PL, Bauman JL. Propafenone: a novel type Ic antiarrhythmic agent. Drug Intell Clin Pharm. 1989;23:196-203.

Quinidine

Kessler KM, Perez GO. Decreased quinidine plasma protein binding during hemodialysis. Clin Pharmacokinet. 1981;30:121-6.

Ochs HR, Greenblatt DJ, Woo E. Clinical pharmacokinetics of quinidine. Clin Pharmacokinet. 1980;5:150-68.

Tocainide

Braun J, Sorgel F, Engelmaier F, Gluth WP, Gebler U. Pharmacokinetics of tocainide in patients with severe renal failure. Eur J Clin Pharmacol. 1985;28:665-70.

Raehl CL, Beirne GJ, Moorthy AV, Patel AK. Tocainide pharmacokinetics during continuous ambulatory peritoneal dialysis. Am J Cardiol. 1987;60: 747-50.

Roden DM, Woosley RL. Tocainide. N Engl J Med. 1986;315:41-5.

Calcium Channel Blockers

Amlodipine

Meredith PA, Elliott HL. Clinical pharmacokinetics of amlodipine. Clin Pharmacokinet. 1992;22:22-31.

Murdoch D, Heel RC. Amlodipine: a review of its pharmacodynamic and pharmacokinetic properties and therapeutic use in cardiovascular disease. Drugs. 1991;41:478-505.

Diltiazem

Chaffman M, Brogden RN. Diltiazem: a review of its pharmacological properties and therapeutic efficacy. Drugs. 1985;29:387-454.

Felodipine

Burr T, Larsson R, Regardh C, Aberg J. Pharmacokinetics of felodipine in chronic hemodialysis patients. J Clin Pharmacokinet. 1991;31:709-13.

Edgar B, Regardh CG, Attman PO, Aurell M, Herlitz H, Johnson G. Pharmacokinetics of felodipine in patients with impaired renal function. Br J Clin Pharmacol. 1989;27:67-74.

Todd PA, Faulds D. Felodipine: a review of the pharmacology and therapeutic use of the extended release formulation in cardiovascular disorders. Drugs. 1992;44:251-77.

Isradipine

Chandler MH, Schran HF, Cutler RE, Smith AJ, Gonasun LM, Blouin RA. The effects of renal function on the disposition of isradipine. J Clin Pharmacol. 1988;28:1076-80.

Fitton A, Benfield P. Isradipine. A review of its pharmacodynamic and pharmacokinetic properties and therapeutic use in cardiovascular disease. Drugs. 1990;40:31-74.

Schonholzer K, Marone C. Pharmacokinetics and dialysability of isradipine in chronic haemodialysis patients. Eur J Clin Pharmacol. 1991;42:231-3.

Nicardipine

Ahmed JH, Grant AC, Rodger RS, Murray G, Elliott H. Inhibitory effect of uremia on hepatic clearance and metabolism of nicardipine. J Clin Pharmacol. 1991;32:57-62.

Sorkin EM, Clissold SP. Nicardipine: a review of its pharmacodynamic and pharmacokinetic properties, and therapeutic efficacy, in the treatment of angina pectoris, hypertension and related cardiovascular disorders. Drugs. 1987;33:296-345.

Nifedipine

Kleinbloesem CH, Van Brummelen P, Woittiez AJ, Faber H, Breimer DD. Influence of haemodialysis on the pharmacokinetics and haemodynamic effects of nifedipine during continuous intravenous infusion. Clin Pharmacokinet. 1986;11:316-22.

Sorkin EM, Clissold SP, Brogden RN. Nifedipine: a review of its pharmacodynamic and pharmacokinetic properties and therapeutic efficacy, in ischaemic heart disease, hypertension and related cardiovascular disorders. Drugs. 1985;30:182-274.

Nimodipine

Langley MS, Sorkin EM. Nimodipine: a review of its pharmacodynamic and pharmakinetic properties, and therapeutic potential in cerebrovascular disease. Drugs. 1989;37:669-99.

Nisoldipine

Boelaert J, Valcke Y, Dammekens H, et al. Pharmacokinetics of nisoldipine in renal dysfunction. Eur J Clin Pharmacol. 1988;34:207-9.

Friedel HA, Sorkin EM. Nisoldipine: a preliminary review of its pharmacodynamic and pharmacokinetic properties, and therapeutic efficacy in the treatment of angina pectoris, hypertension and related cardiovascular disorders. Drugs. 1988;36:682-731.

Nitrendipine

Bortel LV, Bohn R, Mooy J, Schiffers P, Rahn KH. Pharmacokinetics of nitrendipine in terminal renal failure. Eur J Clin Pharmacol. 1989;36:467-71.

Mikus G, Mast V, Fischer C, Machleidt C, Kuhlman U, Eichelbaum M. Pharmacokinetics, bioavailability, metabolism and acute and chronic antihypertensive effects of nitrendipine in patients with chronic renal failure and moderate to severe hypertension. Br J Clin Pharmacol. 1991;31:313-22.

Santiago TM, Lopez LM. Nitrendipine: a new dihydropyridine calcium-channel antagonist for the treatment of hypertension. Drug Intell Clin Pharm. 1990;24:167-75.

Verapamil

McTavish D, Sorkin EM. Verapamil: an updated review of its pharmaco-dynamic and pharmacokinetic properties, and therapeutic use in hyperten-sion. Drugs. 1989;38:19-76.

Pritza DR, Bierman MH, Hammeke MD. Acute toxic effects of sustained release verapamil in chronic renal failure. Arch Intern Med. 1991;151:2081-4.

Cardiac Glycosides

Allen NM, Dunham GD, Sailstad JM, Findlay JW. Clinical and pharmaco-kinetic profiles of digoxin immune FAB in four patients with renal impairment. DICP Ann Pharmacother. 1991;25:1315-20.

Kelly RA, Smith TW. Use and misuse of digitalis blood levels. Heart Disease and Stroke. 1992;1:117-22.

Digitoxin

Graves PE, Fenster PE, MacFarland RT, Marcus FI, Perrier D. Kinetics of digitoxin and the bis- and monodigitoxosides of digitoxigenin in renal insufficiency. Clin Pharmacol Ther. 1984;36:607-12.

Vohringer HF, Rietbrock N. Digitalis therapy in renal failure with special regard to digitoxin. Int J Clin Pharmacol Res. 1981;19:175-84.

Digoxin

Sonnenblick M, Abraham AS, Meshulam Z, Eylath U. Correlation between manifestations of digoxin toxicity and serum digoxin, calcium, potassium, and magnesium concentrations and arterial pH. BMJ. 1983;286:1089-91.

Diuretics

Beermann B, Grind M. Clinical pharmacokinetics of some newer diuretics. Clin Pharmacokinet. 1987;13:254-66.

Brater DC. Pharmacodynamic considerations in the use of diuretics. Annu Rev Pharmacol Toxicol. 1983;23:45-62.

Acetazolamide

Chapron DJ, Gomolin IH, Sweeney KR. Acetazolamide blood concentra-tions are excessive in the elderly propensity for acidosis and relationship to renal function. J Clin Pharmacol. 1989;29:348-53.

Amiloride

George CF. Amiloride handling in renal failure. Br J Clin Pharmacol. 1980;9;94-5.

Spahn H, Reuter K, Mutschler E, Gerok W, Knauf H. Pharmacokinetics of amiloride in renal and hepatic disease. Eur J Clin Pharmacol. 1987;33:493-8.

Bumetanide

Lau HS, Hyneck ML, Berardi RR, Swartz RD, Smith DE. Kinetics, dynamics, and bioavilability of bumetanide in healthy subjects and patients with chronic renal failure. Clin Pharmacol Ther. 1986;39:635-45.

Pentikainen PJ, Pasternack A, Lampainen E, Neuvonen PJ, Pentilla A. Bumetanide kinetics in renal failure. Clin Pharmacol Ther. 1985;37: 582-8.

Ward A, Heel RC. Bumetanide: a review of its pharmacodynamic and pharmacokinetic properties and therapeutic use. Drugs. 1984;28:426-64.

Chlorthalidone

Mulley BA, Parr GD, Rye RM. Pharmacokinetics of chlorthalidone. Eur J Clin Pharmacol. 1980;17:203-7.

Ethacrynic Acid

Pillary VK, Schwartz FD, Aimi K, Kark RM. Transient and permanent deafness following treatment of ethacrynic acid in renal failure. Lancet. 1969;1:77-9.

Furosemide

Boles LL, Shoenwald RD. Furosemide (frusemide): a pharmacokinetic/ pharmacodynamic review (Part 1). Clin Pharmacokinet. 1990;18:381-408.

Riva E, Fossali E, Bettinelli A. Kinetics of furosemide in children with chronic renal failure undergoing regular haemodialysis. Eur J Clin Pharmacol. 1982;21:303-6.

Traeger A, Stein G, Sperschneider H, Keil E. Pharmacokinetic and pharmacodynamic effects of furosemide in patients with impaired renal function. Int J Clin Pharmacol Ther Toxicol. 1984;22:481-6.

Indapamide

Chaffman M, Heel RC, Brogden RN, Speight TM, Avery GS. Indapamide: a review of its pharmacodynamic properties and therapeutic efficacy in hypertension. Drugs. 1984;28:189-235.

Piretanide

Clissold SP, Brogden RN. Piretanide: a preliminary review of its pharmacodynamic and pharmacokinetic properties, and therapeutic efficacy. Drugs. 1985;29:489-530.

Marsh JD, Smith TW. Piretanide: a loop-active diuretic pharmacology, therapeutic efficacy and adverse effects. Pharmacotherapy. 1984;4:170-80.

Walter U, Rockel A, Lahn W, Heidland A, Heptner W. Pharmacokinetics of the loop diuretic piretanide in renal failure. Eur J Clin Pharmacol. 1985; 29:337-43.

Spironolactone

Morris RG, Frewin DB, Taylor WB, Glistak ML, Lehmann DR. The effect of renal and hepatic impairment of spironolactone on digoxin immunoassays. Eur J Clin Pharmacol. 1988;34:233-9.

Skluth HA, Gums JG. Spironolactone: a re-examination. Drug Intell Clin Pharm. 1990;24:52-9.

Thiazides

Niemeyer C, Hasenfub G, Wais U, Knauf H, Schafer-Korting M, Mutschler E. Pharmacokinetics of hydrochlorothiazide in relation to renal function. Eur J Clin Pharmacol. 1983;24:61-5.

Torasemide

Torasemide. A review of its pharmacological properties and therapeutic potential drugs. 1991;41:81-103.

Triamterene

Triamterene and the kidney (Editorial). Lancet. 1986;1:424.

Fairley KF, Woo KT, Birch DF, Leaker BR, Ratnaike S. Triamterene-induced crystalluria and cylinduria: clinical and experimental studies. Clin Nephrol. 1986;26:169-73.

Miscellaneous Cardiac Drugs

Amrinone

Bottorff MB, Rutledge DR, Pieper JA. Evaluation of intravenous amrinone: the first of a new class of positive inotropic agents with vasodilator properties. Pharmacotherapy. 1984;5:227-36.

Dobutamine

Lawless CE, Loeb HS. Pharmacokinetics and pharmacodynamics of Dobutamine. In: Chatterjee ED, ed. Dobutamine. New York: NCM Publishers Inc.; 1989:33-47.

Majerus TC, Dasta JF, Bauman JL, Danziger LH, Ruffolo RR. Dobutamine: ten years later. Pharmacotherapy. 1989;9:245-59.

Milrinone

Larsson R, Liedholm H, Andersson KE, Keane MA, Henry G. Pharmacokinetics and effects on blood pressure of a single oral dose of milrinone in healthy subjects and in patients with renal impairment. Eur J Clin Pharmacol. 1986;29:549-53.

Young RA, Ward A. Milrinone: a preliminary review of its pharmacological properties and therapeutic use. Drugs. 1988;36:158-92.

Nitrates

Evers J, Bonn R, Boertz A, Cawello W, Dickmans HA, Weib M. Pharmacokinetics of isosorbide dinitrate, isosorbide-2-nitrate and isosorbide-5-
nitrate in renal insufficiency after repeated oral dosage. Klin Wochenschr.
1989;67:342-8.

Fung HL. Pharmacokinetics and pharmacodynamics of organic nitrates. Am
J Cardiol. 1987;60:4H-9H.

Todd PA, Goa KL, Langtry HD. Transdermal nitroglycerin (glyceryl tri-
nitrate): a review of its pharmacology and therapeutic use. Drugs. 1990;40:
880-902.

Sedatives, Hypnotics, Drugs Used in Psychiatry

Antidepressants

Cole JO, Bodkin JA. Antidepressant drug side effects [Review]. J Clin
Psychiatry. 1990;51(Suppl):21-6.

Devane CL. Pharmacokinetics of the selective serotonin reuptake inhibitors
[Review]. J Clin Psychiatry. 1992;53(Suppl):13-20.

Elliot-Baker SJ, Singh BS. What has happened to the new antidepressant
drugs [Review]. Med J Aust. 1990;152:150-3.

Potter WZ, Manji HK. Antidepressants, metabolites and apparent drug
resistance [Review]. Clin Neuropharmacol. 1990;13(Suppl 1):S45-53.

Amoxapine (Ascendin)

Calvo B, Garcia MJ, Pedraz JL, Marino EL, Dominquez-Gil A. Pharmacokinetics of amoxapine and its active metabolites. Int J Clin Pharmacol
Ther Toxicol. 1985;23:180-5.

Bupropion (Wellbutren)

Coccaro EF, Siever CJ. Second generation anti-depressants: a comparative
review [Review]. J Clin Pharmacol. 1985;25:241-60.

Goodnick PJ. Pharmacokinetics of second generation antidepressants:
bupropion. Psychopharmacol Bull. 1991;27:513-9.

Laizure SC, Devane CL, Stewart JJ, Demmisse CS, Lai AA. Pharmacokinetics of bupropion and its major basic metabolite in normal subjects after
single dose. Clin Pharmacol Ther. 1985;38:586-9.

Posner J, Bye A, Dean K, Peck AW, Whiteman PD. Disposition of bupropion
and its metabolism in healthy male volunteers after single and multiple
doses. Eur J Clin Pharmacol. 1985;29:97-103.

Suckow RF, Smith TM, Permual AS, Cooper TB. Pharmacokinetics of
bupropion and metabolites in plasma and brain of rats, mice, and guinea
pigs. Drug Metab Dispos. 1986;14:692-7.

Welch RM, Lai AA, Schroeder DH. Pharmacological significance of the
species differences in bupropion metabolism. Xenobiotica. 1987;17:
287-98.

Fluoxetine

Benfield P, Heel RC, Lewis SP. Fluoxetine: a review of its pharmacodynamic and pharmacokinetic properties, and therapeutic efficacy in depressive illness [Review]. Drugs. 1986;32:481-508.

Ciraulo DA, Shader RI. Fluoxetine drug–drug interactions: I. Antidepressants and antipsychotics. J Clin Psychopharmacol 1990;10:48-50.

Ciraulo DA, Shader RI. Fluoxetine drug–drug interactions II. J Clin Psychopharmacol. 1990;10:213-7.

Goodnick PJ. Pharmacokinetics of second generation antidepressants: fluoxetine. Psychopharmacol Bull. 1991;27:503-12.

Lemberger L, Bergstrom RF, Wolen RL, Farid NA, Enis GG, Aronoff GR. Fluoxetine: clinical pharmacology and physiologic disposition. J Clin Psychiatry. 1985;46:14-9.

Lemberger L, Rowe H, Bosomworth JC, Tenbarge JB, Bergstrom RF. The effect of fluoxetine on the pharmacokinetics and psychomotor responses of diazepam. Clin Pharmacol Ther. 1988;43:412-9.

Saletu B, Grunberger J. Classification and determination of cerebral bioavailability of fluoxetine: pharmacokinetic, pharmaco-EEG and psychometric analysis. J Clin Psychiatry. 1985;46:45-52.

Stark P, Fuller RW, Wong DT. The pharmacologic profile of fluoxetine. J Clin Psychiatry. 1985;46:7-13.

Barbiturates

Browne TR. The pharmacokinetics of agents used to treat status epilepticus [Review]. Neurology. 1990;40(Suppl 2):28-32.

Hexobarbital

Baumann P. New aspects in research on blood levels and bioavailability of antidepressants. Psychopathology. 1986;19(Suppl 2):79-84.

Breimer DD, Honhoff C, Zilly W, Richter E, Vanrossum JM. Pharmacokinetics of hexobarbital in plasma of man after intravenous infusion. J Pharmacokinet Biopharm. 1975;3:1-11.

Heinemeyer G, Gramm HJ, Singen W, Dennhardt R, Roots I. Kinetics of hexobarbital and dipyrone in critical care patients receiving high dose pentobarbital. Eur J Clin Pharmacol. 1987;32:273-7.

Sawada Y, Hanano M, Sugiyama Y, Iga T. Prediction of the disposition of nine weakly acidic and six weakly basic drugs in humans from pharmacokinetic parameters in rats [Review]. J Pharmacokinet Biopharm. 1985;13:477-94.

Van der Graff M, Vermeulen NP, Heij P, Boeijinga JK, Breimer DD. Pharmacokinetics of orally administered hexobarbital in plasma and saliva of healthy subjects. Biopharm Drug Dispos. 1986;7:265-72.

Pentobarbital

Wermeling D, Record K, Bell R, Porter W, Blouin R. Hemodialysis clearance of pentobarbital during continuous infusion. Ther Drug Monit. 1985;7:485-7.

Phenobarbital

Chow-Tung E, Lau AH, Vidyasagar D, John EG. Effect of peritoneal dialysis on serum concentrations of three drugs commonly used in pediatric patients. Dev Pharmacol Ther. 1985;8:85-95.

Gillespie WR, Veng-Pederson P, Berg MJ, Schottelius DD. Linear systems approach to the analysis of an induced drug removal process: phenobarbital removal by oral activated charcoal. J Pharmacokinet Biopharm. 1986;14:19-28.

Lau AH, Chow-Tung E, Assadi FK, Fornell L, John E. Effect of ultrafiltration on peritoneal dialysis drug clearances. Pharmacology. 1985;31:284-8.

Melten JW, Wittebrood AJ, Willems HJ, Faber GH, Wemer J, Faber DB. Comparison of equilibrium dialysis, ultrafiltration, and gel permeation chromatography for the determination of free fractions of phenobarbital and phenytoin. J Pharm Sci. 1985;74:692-6.

Mofenson HC, Caraccio TR, Greensher J, Dagostino R, Rossi A. Gastrointestinal dialysis with activated charcoal and cathartic in the treatment of adolescent intoxications. Clin Pediatr. 1985;24:678-84.

Porter RS, Baker EB. Drug clearance by diarrhea induction. Am J Emerg Med. 1985;3:182-6.

Sedman AJ, Molitoris BA, Nakata LM, Gal J. Therapeutic drug monitoring in patients with chronic renal failure: evaluation of the Abbott TD drug assay system. Am J Nephrol. 1986;6:132-4.

Shihab-Eldeen AA, Peck GE, Ash SR, Kaufman G. Evaluation of the sorbent suspension reciprocating dialyser in the treatment of overdose of paracetamol and phenobarbitone. J Pharm Pharmacol. 1988;40:381-7.

Secobarbital

Valentine JL, Hunter S. INTRAV and ORAL: basic interactive computer programs for estimating pharmacokinetic parameters. J Pharm Sci. 1985;74:113-9.

Benzodiazepines

Gaudreault P, Guay J, Thivierge RL, Verdy I. Benzodiazepine poisoning: clinical and pharmacological considerations and treatment [Review]. Drug Saf. 1991;6:247-65.

Greenblatt DJ. Pharmacokinetics and pharmacodynamics [Review]. Hosp Pract. 1990;25(Suppl 2):9-15.

Greenblatt DJ. Benzodiazepine hypnotics: sorting the pharmacokinetic facts [Review]. J Clin Psychiatry. 1991;52(Suppl):4-10.

Trelman DM. Pharmacokinetics and clinical use of benzodiazepines in the management of status epilepticus [Review]. Epilepsia. 1989;30(Suppl 2):S4-10.

Alprazolam

Ciraulo DA, Barnhill JG, Boxenbaum HG, Greenblatt DJ, Smith RB. Pharmacokinetics and clinical effects of alprazolam following single and multiple oral doses in patients with panic disorder. J Clin Pharmacol. 1986;26:292-8.

Devane CL, Ware MR, Lydlard RB. Pharmacokinetics, pharmacodynamics and treatment issues for benzodiazepines: alprazolam, adinazolam and clonazepam. Psychopharmacol Bull. 1991;27:463-73.

Ellinwood EH Jr, Heatherly DG, Nikaido AM, Bjornsson TD, Kilts C. Comparative pharmacokinetics and pharmacodynamics of lorazepam, alprazolam and diazepam. Psychopharmacology (Berlin). 1985;86:392-9.

Greenblatt DJ, Harmatz JS, Dorsey C, Shader RI. Comparative single dose kinetics and dynamics of lorazepam, alprazolam, prazepam and placebo. Clin Pharmacol Ther. 1988;44:326-34.

Norman TR, Burrows GD, McIntyre IM. Pharmacokinetic and pharmacodynamic effects of a single nocturnal dose of alprazolam. Int Clin Psychopharmacol. 1990;5:111-7.

Ochs HR, Greenblatt DJ, Labedzki L, Smith RB. Alprazolam kinetics in patients with renal insufficiency. J Clin Psychopharmacol. 1986;6:292-4.

Scavone JM, Greenblatt DJ, Shader RI. Alprazolam kinetics following sublingual and oral administration. J Clin Psychopharmacol. 1987;7:332-4.

Schmith VD, Piraino B, Smith RB, Kroboth PD. Alprazolam in end-stage renal disease: I. Pharmacokinetics. J Clin Pharmacol. 1991;31:571-9.

Smith RB, Kroboth PD. Influence of dosing regimen on alprazolam and metabolite serum concentrations and tolerance to sedative and psychomotor effects. Psychopharmacology (Berlin). 1987;93:105-12.

Smith RB, Kroboth PD, Vanderlugt JT, Phillips JP, Juhl RP. Pharmacokinetics and pharmacodynamics of alprazolam after oral and IV administration. Psychopharmacology (Berlin). 1984;84:452-6.

Talmud J, Straughan JL, Robins AH. Alprazolam: a new triazolobenzodiazepine. S Afr Med J. 1984;66:297-8.

Chlorazepate (Tranxene)

Deguay R. Efficacy and kinetics of chlorazepate administered to anxious patients in a single daily dose. Can J Psychiatry. 1985;30:414-7.

Chlordiazepoxide (Librium)

Barclay AM. Psychotropic drugs in the elderly: selection of the appropriate agent. Postgrad Med. 1985;77:153-7, 160-2.

Clonazepam (Clonapin)

Andre M, Boutray MJ, Dubruc C, et al. Clonazepam pharmacokinetics and therapeutic efficacy in neonatal seizures. Eur J Clin Pharmacol. 1986;30:585-9.

Faingold CL, Browning RA. Mechanisms of anticonvulsant drug action: II. Drugs primarily used for absence epilepsy [Review]. Eur J Pediatr. 1987;146:8-14.

Diazepam (Valium)

Greenblatt DJ, Harmatz JS, Friedman H, Looniskar A, Shader RI. A large-sample study of diazepam pharmacokinetics. Ther Drug Monit. 1989;11:652-7.

Vanholder R, Van-Landschoot N, De-Smet R, Schoots A, Ringoir S. Drug protein binding in chronic renal failure: evaluation of nine drugs. Kidney Int. 1099;33:996-1004.

Estazolam

Gustavson LE, Carrigan PJ. The clinical pharmacokinetics of a single dose of estazolam. Am J Med. 1990;88(3A):2S-5S.

Flurazepam (Dalmane)

Cook PJ. Benzodiazepine hypnotics in the elderly. Acta Psychiatr Scand Suppl. 1986;332:149-58.

Greenblatt DJ, Harmatz JS, Engelhardt N, Shader RI. Pharmacokinetic determinants of dynamic differences among three benzodiazepine hypnotics: flurazepam, temazepam, and triazolam. Arch Gen Psychiatry. 1989;46:326-32.

Miller LG, Greenblatt DJ, Abernethy DR, et al. Kinetics, brain uptake, and receptor binding characteristics of flurazepam and its metabolites. Psychopharmacology (Berlin). 1988;94:386-91.

Lorazepam (Ativan)

Greenblatt DJ, Harmatz JS, Dorsey C, Shader RI. Comparative single-dose kinetics and dynamics of lorazepam, alprazolam, prazepam, and placebo. Clin Pharmacol Ther. 1988;44:326-34.

Greenblatt DJ, Ehrenberg BL, Gunderman J, et al. Kinetic and dynamic study of intravenous lorazepam: comparison with intravenous diazepam. J Pharmacol Exp Ther 1989;250:134-40.

Midazolam

Bell DM, Richards G, Phillon S, et al. A comparative pharmacokinetic study of intravenous and intramuscular midazolam in patients with epilepsy. Epilepsy Res. 1991;10:183-90.

Castelden CM, Allen JG, Altman J, St.-John-Smith P. A comparison of oral midazolam, nitrazepam and placebo in young and elderly subjects. Eur J Clin Pharmacol. 1987;32:253-7.

Crevat-Pisano P, Dragna S, Granthil C, Coassolo P, Cano JP, Francois G. Plasma concentrations and pharmacokinetics of midazolam during anaesthesia. J Pharm Pharmacol. 1986;38:578-82.

Frye-Kryder S. Midazolam: a new benzodiazepine. AANA J. 1987;55:121-5.

Holazo AA, Winkler MB, Patel IH. Effects of age, gender and oral contraceptives on intramuscular midazolam pharmacokinetics. J Clin Pharmacol. 1988;28:1040-5.

Langlois S, Kreeft JH, Chouinard G, Ross-Chouinard A, East S, Ogilvie RI. Midazolam: kinetics and effects on memory, sensorium, and haemodynamics. Br J Clin Pharmacol. 1987;23:273-8.

Persson P, Nilsson A, Hartvig P, Tamsen A. Pharmacokinetics of midazolam in total IV anaesthesia. Br J Anaesth. 1987;59:548-56.

Raeder JC, Nilsen OG, Hole A. Pharmacokinetics of midazolam and alfentanil in outpatient general anesthesia: a study with concomitant thiopentole, flumazenil or placebo administration. Acta Anaesthesiol Scand. 1988;32:467-72.

Nitrazepam

Castelden CM, Allen JG, Altman J, St.-John-Smith P. A comparison of oral midazolam, nitrazepam and placebo in young and elderly subjects. Eur J Clin Pharmacol. 1987;32:253-7.

Cook PJ. Benzodiazepine hypnotics in the elderly. Acta Psychiatr Scand Suppl. 1986;332:149-58.

Jochemsen R, Breimer DD. Pharmacokinetics of temazepam compared with other benzodiazepine hypnotics: some clinical consequences. Acta Psychiatr Scand Suppl. 1986;332:20-31.

Oxazepam (Serax)

Aso Y, Yoshioka S, Shibazaki T, Uchiyama M. The kinetics of the racemization of oxazepam in aqueous solution. Chem Pharm Bull (Tokyo). 1988;36: 1834-40.

Ayd FJ Jr. Oxazepam: update 1989. Int Clin Psychopharmacol. 1990;5:1-15.

Sonne J, Loft S, Dossing M, et al. Bioavailability and pharmacokinetics of oxazepam. Eur J Clin Pharmacol. 1988;35:385-9.

Prazepam

Greenblatt DJ, Harmatz JS, Dorsey C, Shader RI. Comparative single-dose kinetics and dynamics of lorazepam, alprazolam, prazepam, and placebo. Clin Pharmacol Ther. 1988;44:326-34.

Quazepam

Hilbert JM, Battista D. Quazepam and flurazepam: differential pharmacokinetic and pharmacodynamic characteristics. J Clin Psychiatry. 1991;52: 21-6.

Kales A. Quazepam: hypnotic efficacy and side effects. Pharmacotherapy. 1990;10:2-10.

Temazepam (Restoril)

Greenblatt DJ, Harmatz JS, Engelhardt N, Shader RI. Pharmacokinetic determinants of dynamic differences among three benzodiazepine hypnotics: flurazepam, temazepam, and triazolam. Arch Gen Psychiatry. 1989;46: 326-32.

Jochemsen R, Breimer DD. Pharmacokinetics of temazepam compared with other benzodiazepine hypnotics: some clinical consequences. Acta Psychiatr Scand Suppl. 1986;332:20-31.

Klem K, Murray GR, Laake K. Pharmacokinetics of temazepam in geriatric patients. Eur J Clin Pharmacol. 1986;30:745-7.

Krobath PD, Smith RB, Rault R, et al. Effects of end-stage renal disease and aluminum hydroxide on temazepam kinetics. Clin Pharmacol Ther. 1985;37: 453-9.

Triazolam (Halcion)

Ellinwood EH Jr, Nikaido AM, Heatherly DG. Comparative pharmacodynamics of benzodiazepines. Psychopharmacol Ser. 1987;3:77-82.

Friedman H, Greenblatt DJ, Burstein ES, Scavone JM, Harmatz JS, Shader RI. Triazolam kinetics: interaction with cimetidine, propranolol, and the combination. J Clin Pharmacol. 1988;28:228-33.

Friedman H, Greenblatt DJ, Burstein ES, Harmatz JS, Shader RI. Population study of triazolam pharmacokinetics. Br J Clin Pharmacol. 1986;22: 639-42.

Greenblatt DJ, Harmatz JS, Engelhardt N, Shader RI. Pharmacokinetic determinants of dynamic differences among three benzodiazepine hypnotics: flurazepam, temazepam, and triazolam. Arch Gen Psychiatry. 1989;46: 326-32.

Jochemsen R, Breimer DD. Pharmacokinetics of temazepam compared with other benzodiazepine hypnotics: some clinical consequences. Acta Psychiatr Scand Suppl. 1986;332:20-31.

Kroboth PD, Smith RB, Silver MR, et al. Effects of end stage renal disease and aluminium hydroxide on triazolam pharmacokinetics. Br J Clin Pharmacol. 1985;19:839-42.

Smith RB, Kroboth PD, Varner PD. Pharmacodynamics of triazolam after intravenous administration. J Clin Pharmacol. 1987;27:971-9.

Benzodiazepine Antagonist

Flumazenil

Brogden RN, Goa KL. Flumazenil: a reappraisal of its pharmacological properties and therapeutic efficacy as a benzodiazepine antagonist. Drugs. 1991;42:1061-89.

Karavokiros KA, Tsipis GB. Flumazenil: a benzodiazepine antagonist. DICP. 1990;24:976-81.

Vetey SR, Bosse GM, Boyer MJ, Hoffman JR. Flumazenil: a new benzodiazepine antagonist. Ann Emerg Med. 1991;20:181-8.

Miscellaneous Agents

Buspirone

Caccia S, Vigano GL, Mingardi G, et al. Clinical pharmacokinetics of oral buspirone in patients with impaired renal function. Clin Pharmacokinet. 1988;14:171-7.

Dommisse CE, Devane CL. Buspirone: a new type of anxiolytic [Review]. Drug Intell Clin Pharm. 1985;19:624-8.

Eison AS, Temple DL. Buspirone: review of its pharmacology and current perspectives on its mechanisms of action. Am J Med. 1986;80:1-9.

Gammans RE, Mayol RJ, Labudde JA. Metabolism and disposition of buspirone. Am J Med. 1986;80:41-51.

Goa KL, Ward A. Buspirone: a preliminary review of its pharmacological properties and therapeutic efficacy as an anxiolytic [Review]. Drugs. 1986;32:114-29.

Gulyassy PF, Depner TA. Impaired binding of drugs and endogenous ligands in renal diseases. Am J Kidney Dis. 1983;2:578-601.

Ethchlorvynol

Forycki Z, Martens F, Thalhofer S, Ibe K. Tranquilizers, analgesic and anti-depressants in patients treated with hemodialysis. Blood Purif. 1985;3: 109-19.

Yell RP. Ethchlorvynol overdose. Am J Emerg Med. 1990;8:246-50.

Haloperidol

Fruemming JS, Lam YH, Jann MW, Davis CM. Pharmacokinetics of halo-peridol. Clin Pharmacokinet. 1989;17:396-423.

Lithium Carbonate

Arancibia A, Corvalan F, Mella F, Concha L. Absorption and disposition kinetics of lithium carbonate following administration of conventional and controlled release formulations. Int J Clin Pharmacol Ther Toxicol. 1986; 24:240-5.

Hardy BG, Shulman KI, Mackenzie SE, Kutcher SP, Silverberg JD. Pharmacokinetics of lithium in the elderly. J Clin Psychopharmacol. 1987; 7:153-8.

Luisier PA, Schultz P, Dick P. The pharmacokinetics of lithium in normal humans: expected and unexpected observations in view of basic kinetic principles. Pharmacopsychiatry. 1987;20:232-4.

Shelley RK, Silverstone T. Single dose pharmacokinetics of 5 formulations of lithium: a controlled comparison in healthy subjects. Int Clin Psycho-pharmacol. 1986;1:324-31.

Thornhill DP. Serum levels and pharmacokinetics of ordinary and sustained-release lithium carbonate in manic patients during chronic dosage. Int J Clin Pharmacol Ther Toxicol. 1986;24:257-61.

Meprobamate

Hassan E. Treatment of meprobamate overdose with repeated oral doses of activated charcoal. Ann Emerg Med. 1986;15:73-6.

Jacobsen D, Wiik-Larsen E, Saltvedt E, Bredesen JE. Meprobamate kinet-ics during and after terminated hemoperfusion in acute intoxications. J Toxicol Clin Toxicol. 1987;25:317-31.

Phenothiazines

Chlorpromazine

Indraprarsit S, Sooksriwongse C. Effect of chlorpromazine on peritoneal clearances. Nephron. 1985;40:341-3.

Verbeeck RK, Cardinal JA. Plasma protein binding of salicylic acid, phenytoin, chlorpromazine, propranolol and pethidine using equilibrium dialysis and ultracentrifugation. Arzneimittelforschung. 1985;35:903-6.

Promethazine

Stavchansky S, Wallace JE, Geary R, Hecht G, Robb CA, Wu P. Bioequivalance and pharmacokinetic profile of promethazine hydrochloride suppositories in humans. J Pharm Sci. 1987;76:441-5.

Tricyclic Antidepressants

Sallee FR, Pollock BG. Clinical pharmacokinetics of imipramine and desipramine. Clin Pharmacokinet. 1990;18:346-64.

Amitriptyline

Eap CB, Cuendet C, Baumann P. Selectivity in the binding of psychotropic drugs to the variants of alpha-1 acid glycoprotein. Naunyn-Schmiedebergs Arch Pharmacol. 1988;337:220-4.

Levitt MA, Sullivan JB Jr, Owens SM, Burnham L, Finley PR. Amitriptyline plasma protein binding: effect of plasma pH and relevance to clinical overdose. Am J Emerg Med. 1986;4:121-5.

Tassett JJ, Singh S, Pesce AJ. Evaluation of amitriptyline pharmacokinetics during peritoneal dialysis. Ther Drug Monit. 1985;7:255-7.

Desipramine

Kennedy SH, Craven JL, Roin GM. Major depression in renal dialysis patients: an open trial of antidepressant therapy. J Clin Psychiatry. 1989;50: 60-3.

Doxepin

Coccaro EF, Siever LJ. Second generation antidepressants: a comparative review [Review]. J Clin Pharmacol. 1985;25:241-60.

Joyce PR, Sharman JR. Doxepin plasma concentrations in clinical practice: could there be a pharmacokinetic explanation for low concentrations? Clin Pharmacokinet. 1985;10:365-70.

Scheinin M, Virtanen R, Pisalo E. Effect of single and repeated doses of activated charcoal on the pharmacokinetics of doxepin. Int J Clin Pharmacol Ther Toxicol. 1985;23:38-42.

Sutherland DL, Remillard AJ, Haight KR, Brown MA, Old L. The influence of cimetidine versus ranitidine on doxepin pharmacokinetics. Eur J Clin Pharmacol. 1987;32:159-64.

Wecker MT, Woodworth JR, Amsel LP, Hinsvark ON, Rotenberg KS. Pharmacokinetic evaluation of two doxepin products. Clin Ther. 1986;8: 342-7.

El-Yazigi A, Chaleby K. Steady-state kinetics of doxepin and imipramine in Saudi patients with interethnic comparison [Review]. Psychopharmacology (Berlin). 1988;95:63-7.

Imipramine

Bickel MH, Raaflaub RM, Hellmuller M, Stauffer EJ. Characterization of drug distribution and binding competition by two-chamber and multi-chamber distribution dialysis. J Pharm Sci. 1987;76:68-74.

Lieberman JA, Cooper TB, Suckow RF, et al. Tricyclic antidepressant and metabolite levels in chronic renal failure. Clin Pharmacol Ther. 1985;37: 301-7.

Lithium Carbonate

Goodnick PJ, Schorr-Cain CB. Lithium pharmacokinetics. Psychopharmacol Bull. 1991;27:475-91.

Nortriptyline

El-Yazigi A, Chaleby K. Steady-state concentrations of amitriptyline and its metabolite nortriptyline in Saudi patients. Ther Drug Monit. 1987;9:6-10.

Kumar V, Smith RC, Reed K, Leelavathi DE. Plasma levels and effects of nortriptyline in geriatric depressed patients. Acta Psychiatr Scand. 1987; 75:20-8.

Sirdal L, Lundgren TI, Bessessen A, Sager G. Distribution of nortriptyline in human blood: effects of temperature, pH, and drug concentration. Ther Drug Monit. 1987;9:67-71.

Analgesics

Narcotics and Narcotic Antagonists

Alfentanil

Chauvin M, Lebrault C, Levron JC, Duvaldestin P. Pharmacokinetics of alfentanil in chronic renal failure. Anesth Analg. 1987;66:53-6.

Davis PJ, Cook DR. Clinical pharmacokinetics of the newer IV anesthetic agents. Clin Pharmacokinet. 1986;11:18-35.

Mather LE. Opioid pharmacokinetics in relation to their effects [Review]. Anaesth Intensive Care. 1987;15:15-22.

Meistelman C, Saint-Maurice C, Lepaul M, Levron JC, Loose JP, MacGee K. A comparison of alfentanil pharmacokinetics in children and adults. Anesthesiology. 1987;66:13-6.

O'Connor M, Prys-Roberts C, Sear JW. Alfentanil infusions: relationship between pharmacokinetics and pharmacodynamics in man. Eur J Anaesthesiol. 1987;4:187-96.

Persson MP, Nilsson A, Hartvig P. Pharmacokinetics of alfentanil in total I.V. anaesthesia. Br J Anaesth. 1988;60:755-61.

Raeder JC, Nilsen OG, Hole A. Pharmacokinetics of midazolam and alfentanil in outpatient general anesthesia: a study with concomitant thiopentone, flumazenil or placebo administration. Acta Anaesthesiol Scand. 1988;32: 467-72.

Sitar DS, Duke PC, Benthuysen JL, Sanford TJ, Smith NT. Aging and alfentanil disposition in healthy volunteers and surgical patients. Can J Anaesth. 1989;36:149-54.

Stanski DR. Narcotic pharmacokinetics and dynamics: the basis of infusion applications [Review]. Anaesth Intensive Care. 1987;15:23-6.

VanPeer A. Review of clinical pharmacokinetics of alfentanil. Acta Anaesthesiol Belg. 1984;35(Suppl):261-3.

VanPeer A, Vercauteren M, Noorduin H, Woestenborghs R, Heykants J. Alfentanil kinetics in renal insufficiency. Eur J Clin Pharmacol. 1986;30: 245-7.

Waud BE, Waud DR. Dose response curves and pharmacokinetics. Anesthesiology. 1986;65:355-8.

Butorphanol

Ramsey R, Higbee M, Maesner J, Wood J. Influence of age on the pharmacokinetics of butorphanol. Acute Care. 1986;12(Suppl 1):8-16.

Codeine

Bodd E. Pharmacokinetic interaction between substances with opioid effects and ethanol. Pharmacol Toxicol. 1987;60(Suppl 2):1-40.

Quiding H, Anderson P, Bondesson U, Boreus LD, Hynning PA. Plasma concentrations of codeine and its metabolite, morphine, after single and repeated oral administration. Eur J Clin Pharmacol. 1986;30:673-7.

Fentanyl

Reilly CS, Wood AJ, Wood M. Variability of fentanyl pharmacokinetics in man: computer predicted plasma concentrations for three intravenous dosage regimens. Anaesthesia. 1985;40:837-43.

Meperidine (Demerol)

Chan K, Tse J, Jennings F, Orme ML. Pharmacokinetics of low-dose intravenous pethidine in patients with renal dysfunction. J Clin Pharmacol. 1987;27:516-22.

Sjostrom S, Hartvig P, Persson MP, Tamsen A. Pharmacokinetics of epidural morphine and meperidine in humans. Anesthesiology. 1987;67: 877-88.

Sjostrom S, Tamsen A, Persson MP, Hartvig P. Pharmacokinetics of intrathecal morphine and meperidine in humans. Anesthesiology. 1987;67: 889-95.

Verbeeck RK, Cardinal JA. Plasma protein binding of salicylic acid, phenytoin, chlorpromazine, propranolol and pethidine using equilibrium dialysis and ultracentrifugation. Arzneimittelforschung. 1985;35:903-6.

Methadone

Garrett ER, Derendorf H, Mattha AG. Pharmacokinetics of morphine and its surrogates: VII. High-performance liquid chromatographic analyses and pharmacokinetics of methadone and its derived metabolites in dogs. J Pharm Sci. 1985;74:1203-14.

Inturrisi CE, Colburn WA, Kaiko RF, Houde RW, Foley KM. Pharmacokinetics and pharmacodynamics of methadone in patients with chronic pain. Clin Pharmacol Ther. 1987;41:392-401.

Sawe J. High-dose morphine and methadone in cancer patients: clinical pharmacokinetic considerations of oral treatment [Review]. Clin Pharmacokinet. 1986;11:87-106.

Morphine

Chauvin M, Sandouk P, Scherrmann JM, Farinotti R, Strumaza P, Duvaldestin P. Morphine pharmacokinetics in renal failure. Anesthesiology. 1987;66:327-31.

Savarese JJ, Goldenheim PD, Thomas GB, Kaiko RF. Steady-state pharmacokinetics of controlled release oral morphine sulphate in healthy subjects. Clin Pharmacokinet. 1986;11:505-10.

Sawe J. High-dose morphine and methadone in cancer patients. Clinical pharmacokinetic considerations of oral treatment [Review]. Clin Pharmacokinet. 1986;11:87-106.

Sjostrom S, Hartvig P, Persson MP, Tamsen A. Pharmacokinetics of epidural morphine and meperidine in humans. Anesthesiology. 1987;67:877-88.

Sjostrom S, Tamsen A, Persson MP, Hartvig P. Pharmacokinetics of intrathecal morphine and meperidine in humans. Anesthesiology. 1987;67:889-95.

Pentazocine (Talwin)

Forycki Z, Martens F, Thalhofer S, Ibe K. Tranquilizers, analgesics and antidepressants in patients treated with hemodialysis [Review]. Blood Purif. 1985;3:109-19.

Mather LE. Opioid pharmacokinetics in relation to their effects. Anaesth Intensive Care. 1987;15:15-22.

Ritschel WA, Hoffmann KA, Willig JL, Frederick KA, Wetzelsberger N. The effect of age on the pharmacokinetics of pentazocine. Methods Find Exp Clin Pharmacol. 1986;8:497-503.

Sawada Y, Hanano M, Sugiyama Y, Iga T. Prediction of the disposition of nine weakly acidic and six weakly basic drugs in humans from pharmacokinetic parameters in rats [Review]. J Pharmacokinet Biopharm. 1985;13:477-92.

Yeh SY, Todd GD, Johnson RE, Gorodetzky CW, Lange WR. The pharmacokinetics of pentazocine and tripelennamine. Clin Pharmacol Ther. 1986;39:669-76.

Propoxyphene (Darvon)

Colburn WA, Inturrisi CE. Propoxyphene: accumulation or altered kinetics? [Letter]. Eur J Clin Pharmacol. 1985;28:725-6.

Sufentanil

Davis PJ, Stiller RL, Cook DR, Brandom RW, Davin-Robinson KA. Pharmacokinetics of sufentanil in adolescent patients with chronic renal failure. Anesth Analg. 1988;67:268-71.

Fyman PN, Reynolds JR, Moser F, Avitable M, Casthely PA, Butt K. Pharmacokinetics of sufentanil in patients undergoing renal transplantation. Can J Anaesth. 1988;35:312-5.

Wiggum DC, Cork RC, Weldon ST, Gandolfi AJ, Perry DS. Postoperative respiratory depression and elevated sufentanil levels in a patient with chronic renal failure. Anesthesiology. 1985;63:708-10.

Non-narcotic Drugs

Acetaminophen

Clissold SP. Paracetamol and phenacetin. Drugs. 1986;32(Suppl 4):46-59.

Davenport A, Finn R. Paracetamol (acetaminophen) poisoning resulting in acute renal failure with hepatic coma. Nephron. 1988;50:55-6.

Meredith TJ, Vale JA. Non-narcotic analgesics: problems of overdosage. Drugs. 1986;32(Suppl 4):177-205.

Segasothy M, Suleiman AB, Puvaneswary M, Rohana A. Paracetamol: a cause for analgesic nephropathy and end-stage renal disease. Nephron. 1988;50:50-4.

Shihab-Eldeen AA, Peck GE, Ash SR, Kaufman G. Evaluation of the sorbent suspension reciprocating dialyser in the treatment of overdose of paracetamol and phenobarbitone. J Pharm Pharmacol. 1988;40:381-7.

Verbeeck RK, Cardinal JA. Plasma protein binding of salicylic acid, phenytoin, chlorpromazine and pethidine using equilibrium dialysis and ultracentrifugation. Arzneimittelforschung. 1985;35:903-6.

Acetylsalicylic Acid (Aspirin)

Clissold SP. Aspirin and related derivatives of salicylic acid. Drugs. 1986; 32(Suppl 4):8-26.

Grace EM, Amirudin AM, Sweeney GD, Rosenfeld JM, Darke AC, Buchanin WW. Lowering of plasma isoxicam concentrations with acetylsalicylic acid. J Rheumatol. 1986;13:119-21.

Latini R, Cerletti C, Degaeratano G, et al. Comparative bioavailability of aspirin from buffered, enteric coated and plain preparations. Int J Clin Pharmacol Ther Toxicol. 1986;24:313-8.

Mofenson HC, Caraccio TR, Greensher J, D'Agostino R, Rossi A. Gastrointestinal dialysis with activated charcoal and cathartic in treatment of adolescent intoxication. Clin Pediatr (Phila). 1985;24:678-82.

Montgomery PR, Berger LG, Mitenko PA, Sitar DS. Salicylate metabolism: effects of age and sex in adults. Clin Pharmacol Ther. 1986;39:571-6.

Montgomery PR, Sitar DS. Acetylsalicylic acid metabolites in blood and urine after plain and enteric coated tablets. Biopharm Drug Dispos. 1986;7: 21-5.

Needs CJ, Brooks PM. Clinical pharmacokinetics of the salicylates. Clin Pharmacokinet. 1985;10:165-77.

Nitelius E, Melander A, Wahlin-Boll E. Pharmacokinetic interaction of acetylsalicylic acid and dipyridamole. Br J Clin Pharmacol. 1985;19: 379-83.

Miscellaneous Agents

Anticoagulants, Antifibrinolytic and Antiplatelet Agents

Dipyridamole

Fitzgerald GA. Dipyridamole. N Engl J Med. 1987;316:1247-51.

Mahoney G, Wolfram KM, Cochetto D, Bjornsson TD. Dipyridamole kinetics. Clin Pharmacol Ther. 1982;31:330-8.

Heparin

Perry PJ, Herron GR, King JC. Heparin half-life in normal and impaired renal function. Clin Pharmacol Ther. 1974;16:514-9.

Thien AN, Bjornsson J. Heparin elimination in uraemic patients on hemodialysis. Scand J Haematol. 1977;17:29-35.

Indobufen

Savazzi GM, Castiglioni A, Cavatorta A. Effect of renal insufficiency on the pharmacokinetics of indobufen. Curr Therap Res. 1984;36:119-25.

Streptokinase

Grierson DS, Bjornsson TD. Pharmacokinetics of streptokinase in patients based on amidolytic activator complex activity. Clin Pharmacol Ther. 1987;41:304-13.

Sulfinpyrazone

Margulies EH, White AM, Sherry S. Sulfinpyrazone: a review of its pharmacological properties and therapeutic use. Drugs. 1980;20:179-97.

Pedersen AK, Jakobsen P, Kampmann JP, Hansen JM. Clinical pharmacokinetics and potentially important drug interactions of sulfinpyrazone. Clin Pharmacokinet. 1982;7:42-56.

Ticlopidine

Saltiel E, Ward A. Ticlopidine: a review of its pharmacodynamic and pharmacokinetic properties, and therapeutic efficacy in platelet-dependent disease states. Drugs. 1987;34:222-62.

Warfarin

Kelly JG, O'Malley K. Clinical pharmacokinetics of oral anticoagulants. Clin Pharmacokinet. 1979;4:1-15.

Van Peer A, Belparie F, Bogaert M. Warfarin elimination and responsiveness in patients with renal dysfunction. J Clin Pharmacol. 1978;18:84-8.

Anticonvulsants

Carbamazepine

Bertilsson L, Tomson T. Clinical pharmacokinetics and pharmacological effects of carbamazepine and carbamazepine-10,11-epoxide: an update. Clin Pharmacokinet. 1986;11:177-98.

Lee CS, Wang LH, Marbury TC, Bruni J, Peschalski RJ. Hemodialysis clearance and total body elimination of carbamazepine during chronic hemodialysis. Clin Toxicol. 1980;17:429-38.

Ethosuximide

Marbury TC, Lee CS, Perchalski RJ, Wilder BJ. Hemodialysis clearance of ethosuximide in patients with chronic renal disease. Am J Hosp Pharm. 1981;38:1757-60.

Lamotrigine

Cohen AF, Land GS, Breimer DD, Yuen WC, Winton C, Peck AW. Lamotrigine, a new anticonvulsant: pharmacokinetics in normal humans. Clin Pharmacol Ther. 1987;42:535-41.

Phenytoin

Borga O, Hoppel C, Odar-Cederlof I, Garle M. Plasma levels and renal excretion of phenytoin and its metabolites in patients with renal failure. Clin Pharmacol Ther. 1979;26:306-14.

Primidone

Lee CS, Marbury TC, Perchalski RT, Wilder BJ. Pharmacokinetics of primidone elimination by uremic patients. J Clin Pharmacol. 1982;22: 301-8.

Sodium Valproate

Browne TR. Valproic acid. N Engl J Med. 1980;302:661-6.

Zaccara G, Messori A, Moroni F. Clinical pharmacokinetics of valproic acid—1988. Clin Pharmacokinet. 1988;15:367-89.

Vigabatrin

Schechter PJ. Clinical pharmacology of vigabatrin. Br J Clin Pharmacol. 1989;27:19S-22S.

Antihistamines

Histamine H-1 Antagonists

Astemizole

Richards DM, Brogden RN, Heel RC, Speight TM, Avery GS. Astemizole: a review of its pharmacodynamic properties and therapeutic efficacy. Drugs. 1984;28:38-61.

Flunarizine

Holmes B, Brogden RN, Heel RC, Speight TM, Avery GS. Flunarizine: a review of its pharmacodynamic and pharmacokinetic properties and therapeutic use. Drugs. 1984;27:6-44.

Oxatomide

Richards DM, Brogden RN, Heel RC, Speight TM, Avery GS. Oxatomide: a review of its pharmacodynamic properties and therapeutic efficacy. Drugs. 1984;27:210-31.

Terfenadine

Sorkin EM, Heel RC. Terfenadine: a review of its pharmacodynamic properties and therapeutic efficacy. Drugs. 1985;29:34-56.

Histamine H-2 Antagonists

Cimetidine

Larsson R, Norlander B, Bodemar G, Walan A. Steady-state kinetics and dosage requirements of cimetidine in renal failure. Clin Pharmacokinet. 1981;6:316-25.

Somogyi A, Gugler R. Clinical pharmacokinetics of cimetidine. Clin Pharmacokinet. 1983;8:463-95.

Famotidine

Campoli-Richards DM, Clissold SP. Famotidine: pharmacodynamic and pharmacokinetic properties and a preliminary review of its therapeutic use in peptic ulcer disease and Zollinger-Ellison syndrome. Drugs. 1986;32:197-221.

Nizatidine

Price AH, Brogden RN. Nizatidine: a preliminary review of its pharmacodynamic and pharmacokinetic properties, and its therapeutic use in peptic ulcer disease. Drugs. 1988;36:521-39.

Ranitidine

Grant SM, Langtry HD, Brogden RN. Ranitidine: an updated review of its pharmacodynamic and pharmacokinetic properties and therapeutic use in peptic ulcer disease and other allied diseases. Drugs. 1989;37:801-70.

Meffin PJ, Grgurinovich N, Brooks PM, Miners JO, Cochran M, Stranks G. Ranitidine disposition in patients with renal impairment. Br J Clin Pharmacol. 1983;16:731-4.

Antineoplastic Agents

Azathioprine

Bach JF, Dardenne M. The metabolism of azathioprine in renal failure. Transplantation. 1971;12:253-9.

Bleomycin

Bennett JM, Reich SD. Bleomycin. Ann Intern Med. 1979;90:945-8.

Dalgleish AG, Woods RL, Levi JA. Bleomycin pulmonary toxicity: its relationship to renal dysfunction. Med Pediatr Oncol. 1984;12:313-7.

Busulfan

Ehrsson H, Hassan M, Ehrnebo M, Beran M. Busulfan kinetics. Clin Pharmacol Ther. 1983;34:86-9.

Millard RJ. Busulfan haemorrhagic cystitis. Br J Urol. 1978;50:210.

Cisplatin

Blachley JD, Hill JB. Renal and electrolyte disturbances associated with cisplatin. Ann Intern Med. 1981;95:628-32.

Gormley PE, Bull JM, Leroy AF, Cysyk R. Kinetics of cisdichloro-diammineplatinum. Clin Pharmacol Ther. 1979;25:351-7.

Cyclophosphamide

Grochow LB, Colvin M. Clinical pharmacokinetics of cyclophosphamide. Clin Pharmacokinet. 1979;4:380-94.

Kroener J, Green M. Cyclophosphamide dose in renal failure [Letter]. Am J Med. 1978;64:725-6.

Cytarabine

Wan SH, Huffman DH, Azarnoff DL, Hoogstraten B, Larsen WE. Pharmacokinetics of 1-beta-D-arabinofuranosylcytosine in humans. Cancer Res. 1974;34:392-7.

Doxorubicin

Benjamin RS, Riggs CE Jr, Bachur NR. Plasma pharmacokinetics of adriamycin and its metabolites in humans with normal hepatic and renal function. Cancer Res. 1977;37:1416-20.

Speth PA, Van Hoesel QG, Haanen C. Clinical pharmacokinetics of doxorubicin. Clin Pharmacokinet. 1988;15:15-31.

Etoposide

Clark PI, Slevin ML. The clinical pharmacology of etoposide and teniposide.
Clin Pharmacokinet. 1987;12:223-52.
Sinkule JA. Etoposide: a semisynthetic epipodophyllotoxin. Chemistry, pharmacology, pharmacokinetics, adverse effects and use as an antineoplastic
agent. Pharmacotherapy. 1984;4:61-73.

Fluorouracil

Diasio RB, Harris BE. Clinical pharmacology of 5-fluorouracil. Clin Pharmacokinet. 1989;16:215-37.
MacMillan WE, Wolberg WH, Welling PG. Pharmacokinetics of fluoro-
uracil in humans. Cancer Res. 1978;38:3479-82.

Melphalan

Alberts DS, Chang SY, Chen HG, et al. Kinetics of intravenous melphalan.
Clin Pharmacol Ther. 1979;26:73-80.

Methotrexate

Jolivet J, Cowan KH, Curt GA, Clendeninn NJ, Chabner BA. The pharmacol-
ogy and clinical use of methotrexate. N Engl J Med. 1983;309:1094-104.
Shen DD, Azarnoff DL. Clinical pharmacokinetics of methotrexate. Clin
Pharmacokinet. 1978;3:1-13.

Mitomycin C

Den Hartigh J, McVie JG, Van Oort WS, Pinedo HM. Pharmacokinetics of
mitomycin C in humans. Cancer Res. 1983;43:5017-21.
Giroux L, Bettez P, Giroux L. Mitomycin-C nephrotoxicity: a clinico-
pathologic study of 17 cases. Am J Kidney Dis. 1985;6:28-39.

Nitrosoureas

Ellis ME, Weiss RB, Kuperminc M. Nephrotoxicity of lomustine: a case
report and literature review. Cancer Chemother Pharmacol. 1985;15:174-5.
Oliverio VT. Toxicology and pharmacology of the nitrosoureas. Cancer
Chemother Rep. 1973;4:13-20.

Plicamycin

Kennedy BJ. Metabolic and toxic effects of mithramycin during tumor therapy. Am J Med. 1970;49:494-503.

Streptozocin

Hall-Craggs M, Brenner DE, Vigorito RD, Sutherland JC. Acute renal
failure and renal tubular squamous metaplasia following treatment with
streptozocin. Hum Pathol. 1982;13:597-601.

Tamoxifen

Buckley MM, Goa KL. Tamoxifen: a reappraisal of its pharmacodynamic and pharmacokinetic properties, and therapeutic use. Drugs. 1989;37:451-90.

Teniposide

See Etoposide.

Vinblastine

Owellen RJ, Hartke CA, Hains FO. Pharmacokinetics and metabolism of vinblastine in humans. Cancer Res. 1977;37:2597-602.

Vincristine

Owellen RJ, Root MA, Hains FO. Pharmacokinetics of vinblastine and vincristine in humans. Cancer Res. 1977;37:2603-7.

Antiparkinson Agents

Levodopa

Nutt JG, Fellman JH. Pharmacokinetics of levodopa. Clin Neuropharmacol. 1984;7:35-49.

Robertson DR, Wood ND, Everest H, et al. The effect of age on the pharmacokinetics of levodopa administered alone and in the presence of carbidopa. Br J Clin Pharmacol. 1989;28:61-9.

Trihexyphenidyl

Burke RE, Fahn S. Pharmacokinetics of trihexyphenidyl after short-term and long-term administration of dystonic patients. Ann Neurol. 1985;18:35-40.

Antithyroid Drugs

Methimazole

Jansson R, Lindstrom B, Dahlberg PA. Pharmacokinetic properties and bioavailability of methimazole. Clin Pharmacokinet. 1985;10:443-50.

Propylthiouracil

Cooper DS. Antithyroid drugs. N Engl J Med. 1984;311:1353-62.

Arthritis and Gout Agents

Allopurinol

Hande K, Noone RM, Stone WJ. Severe allopurinol toxicity: description and guidelines for prevention in patients with renal insufficiency. Am J Med. 1984;76:47-56.

Murrell GA, Rapeport WG. Clinical pharmacokinetics of allopurinol. Clin Pharmacokinet. 1986;11:343-53.

Auranofin

Chaffman M, Brogden RN, Heel RC, Speight TM, Avery GS. Auranofin: a preliminary review of its pharmacological properties and therapeutic use in rheumatoid arthritis. Drugs. 1984;27:378-424.

Colchicine

Wallace SL, Omokoku B, Ertel NH. Colchicine plasma levels: implications as to pharmacology and mechanisms of action. Am J Med. 1970;48:443-8.

Gold Sodium Thiomalate

Blocka KL, Paulus HE, Furst DE. Clinical pharmacokinetics of oral and injectable gold compounds. Clin Pharmacokinet. 1986;11:133-43.

Lorber A. Monitoring gold plasma levels in rheumatoid arthritis. Clin Pharmacokinet. 1977;2:127-46.

Penicillamine

Bergstrom RJ, Kay DR, Harkcom TM, Wagner JG. Penicillamine kinetics in normal subjects. Clin Pharmacol Ther. 1981;30:404-13.

Lang K. Nephropathy induced by D-penicillamine. Contrib Nephrol. 1978; 10:63-74.

Netter P, Bannwarth B, Pere P, Nicolas A. Clinical pharmacokinetics of D-penicillamine. Clin Pharmacokinet. 1987;13:317-33.

Probenecid

Cunningham RF, Israili ZH, Dayton PG. Clinical pharmacokinetics of probenecid. Clin Pharmacokinet. 1981;6:135-51.

Dayton PG, Perel JM. The metabolism of probenecid in man. Ann N Y Acad Sci. 1971;179:399-402.

Nonsteroidal Anti-inflammatory Drugs

Diclofenac

Todd PA, Sorkin EM. Diclofenac sodium: a reappraisal of its pharmacodynamic and pharmacokinetic properties, and therapeutic efficacy. Drugs. 1988;35:244-85.

Ibuprofen

Albert KS, Gernaat CM. Pharmacokinetics of ibuprofen. Am J Med. 1984;77: 40-6.

Indomethacin

Helleberg L. Clinical pharmacokinetics of indomethacin. Clin Pharmacokinet. 1981;6:245-58.

Stein G, Kunze M, Zaumseil J, Traeger A. Pharmacokinetics of indomethacin and indomethacin metabolites administered continually to patients with healthy or damaged kidneys. Int J Clin Pharmacol Biopharm. 1977;15:470-3.

Isoxicam

Bury RW, Whitworth JA, Saines D, Kincaid-Smith P, Moulds RF. Effect of impairment of renal function on the accumulation and disposition of isoxicam. Eur J Clin Pharmacol. 1985;28:585-8.

Naproxen

Anttila M, Haataja M, Kasanen A. Pharmacokinetics of naproxen in subjects with normal and impaired renal function. Eur J Clin Pharmacol. 1980;18: 263-8.

Phenylbutazone

Aarbakke J. Clinical pharmacokinetics of phenylbutazone. Clin Pharmacokinet. 1978;3:369-80.

Piroxicam

Brogden RN, Heel RC, Speight TM, Avery GS. Piroxicam: a reappraisal of its pharmacology and therapeutic efficacy. Drugs. 1984;28:292-323.

Sulindac

Miller MJ, Bednar MM, McGiff JC. Renal metabolism of sulindac: functional implications. J Pharmacol Exp Ther. 1984;231:449-56.

Tolmetin

Selley ML, Glass J, Triggs EG, Thomas J. Pharmacokinetic studies of tolmetin in man. Clin Pharmacol Ther. 1975;17:599-605.

Bronchodilators

Albuterol

Morgan DJ, Paull JD, Richmond BH, Wilson-Evered E, Ziccone SP. Pharmacokinetics of intravenous and oral salbutamol and its sulphate conjugate. Br J Clin Pharmacol. 1986;22:587-93.

Powell ML, Chung M, Weisberger M, et al. Multiple-dose albuterol kinetics. J Clin Pharmacol. 1986;26:643-6.

Dyphylline

Lee CS, Wang LH, Majeske BL, Marbury TC. Pharmacokinetics of dyphylline elimination by uremic patients. J Pharmacol Exp Ther. 1981; 217:340-4.

Ipratropium

Ensing K, De Zeeuw RA, Nossent GD, Koeter GH, Cornelissen PJ. Pharmacokinetics of ipratropium bromide after single dose inhalation and oral and intravenous administration. Eur J Clin Pharmacol. 1989;36:189-94.

Theophylline

Hendeles L, Massanari M, Weinberger M. Update on the pharmacodynamics and pharmacokinetics of theophylline. Chest. 1985;88(Suppl 2): 103S-11S.

Kradjan WA, Martin TR, Delaney CL, Blair AD, Cutler RE. Effect of hemodialysis on the pharmacokinetics of theophylline in chronic renal failure. Nephron. 1982;32:40-4.

Corticosteroids

Dexamethasone

Brady ME, Sartiano GP, Rosenblum SL, Zaglama NE, Bauguess CT. The pharmacokinetics of single high doses of dexamethasone in cancer patients. Eur J Clin Pharmacol. 1987;32:593-6.

Methylprednisolone

Al-Habet SM, Rogers HJ. Methylprednisolone pharmacokinetics after intravenous and oral administration. Br J Clin Pharmacol. 1989;27:285-90.

Prednisolone and Prednisone

Bergrem H. Pharmacokinetics and protein binding of prednisolone in patients with nephrotic syndrome and patients undergoing hemodialysis. Kidney Int. 1983;23:876-81.

Lefler UF, Fre FJ, Benet LZ. Prednisolone clearance at steady state in man. J Clin Endocrinol Metab. 1982;55:762.

Pickup ME. Clinical pharmacokinetics of prednisone and prednisolone. Clin Pharmacokinet. 1979;4:111-28.

Triamcinolone

Mollmann H, Rohdewald P, Schmidt EW, Salomon V, Derendorf H. Pharmacokinetics of triamcinolone acetonide and its phosphate ester. Eur J Clin Pharmacol. 1985;29:85-9.

Hypoglycemic Agents

Acetohexamide

Baba S, Baba T, Iwanaga T. Effect of acetohexamide (a sulfonylurea hypoglycemia agent) in blood plasma on creatinine assay in clinical laboratory tests. Chem Pharm Bull (Tokyo). 1979;27:139-43.

Chlorpropamide

Taylor JA. Pharmacokinetics and biotransformation of chlorpropamide in man. Clin Pharmacol Ther. 1972;13:710-8.

Gliclazide

Holmes B, Heel RC, Brogden RN, Speight TM, Avery GS. Gliclazide: a preliminary review of its pharmacodynamic properties and therapeutic efficacy in diabetes mellitus. Drugs. 1984;27:301-27.

Glipizide

Lebovitz HE. Glipizide: a second-generation sulfonylurea hypoglycemic agent: pharmacology, pharmacokinetics and clinical use. Pharmacotherapy. 1985;5:63-77.
Wensing G. Topics in clinical pharmacology. Glipizide: an oral hypoglycemic drug. Am J Med Sci. 1989;298:69-71.

Glyburide

Feldman JM. Glyburide: a second-generation sulfonylurea hypoglycemic agent. History, chemistry, metabolism, pharmacokinetics, clinical use and adverse effects. Pharmacotherapy. 1985;5:43-62.

Insulin

Brogden RN, Heel RC. Human insulin: a review of its biological activity, pharmacokinetics and therapeutic use. Drugs. 1987;34:350-71.
Rabkin R, Simon NM, Steinder S, et al. Effect of renal disease on renal uptake and excretion of insulin in man. N Engl J Med. 1970;282:182-7.

Tolbutamide

Nelson E. Rate of metabolism of tolbutamide in test subjects with liver disease or with impaired renal function. Am J Med Sci. 1964;248:657-9.

Hypolipidemic Agents

Bezafibrate

Monk JP, Todd PA. Bezafibrate: a review of its pharmacodynamic and pharmacokinetic properties, and therapeutic use in hyperlipidaemia. Drugs. 1987;33:539-76.

Cholestyramine

Silverberg DS, Iaina A, Reisin E, Rotzak R, Eliahou HE. Cholestyramine in uremic pruritis. Br Med J. 1977;1:752-3.

Clofibrate

Gugler R. Clinical pharmacokinetics of hypolipidaemic drugs. Clin Pharmacokinet. 1978;3:425-39.

Gemfibrozil

Manninen V, Malkonen M, Eisalo A. Gemfibrozil treatment of dyslipidaemias in renal failure with uremia or in the nephrotic syndrome. Res Clin Forums. 1982;4:113-8.

Todd PA, Ward A. Gemfibrozil: a review of its pharmacodynamic and pharmacokinetic properties, and therapeutic use in dyslipidaemia. Drugs. 1988;36:314-39.

Lovastatin

Henwood JM, Heel RC. Lovastatin: a preliminary review of its pharmacodynamic properties and therapeutic use in hyperlipidaemia. Drugs. 1988; 36:429-54.

Nicotinic Acid

Gokal R, Mann JI, Oliver DO, Ledingham JG, Cartes RD. Treatment of hyperlipidemia in patients on chronic hemodialysis. Br Med J. 1978;1:82-3.

Miscellaneous Agents

Acetohydroxamic Acid

Lake KD, Brown DC. New drug therapy for kidney stones: a review of cellulose sodium phosphate, acetohydroxamic acid, and potassium citrate. Drug Intell Clin Pharm. 1985;19:530-9.

Clodronate

Conrad KA, Lee SM. Clodronate kinetics and dynamics. Clin Pharmacol Ther. 1981;30:114-20.

Cyclosporine

Awni WM, Kasiske BL, Heim-Duthoy K, Rao KV. Long-term cyclosporine pharmacokinetic changes in renal transplant recipients: effects of binding and metabolism. Clin Pharmacol Ther. 1989;45:41-8.

Fullath F, Wenk M, Vozeh S, et al. Intravenous cyclosporine kinetics in renal failure. Clin Pharmacol Ther. 1983;34:638-43.

Rodighiero V. Therapeutic drug monitoring of cyclosporine: practical applications and limitations. Clin Pharmacokinet. 1989;16:27-37.

Deferoxamine

Allain P, Mauras Y, Chaleil D, et al. Pharmacokinetics and renal elimination of desferrioxamine and ferrioxamine in healthy subjects and patients with haemochromatosis. Br J Clin Pharmacol. 1987;24:207-12.

Metoclopramide

Bateman DN. Clinical pharmacokinetics of metoclopramide. Clin Pharmacokinet. 1983;8:523-9.

N-Acetylcysteine

Borgstrom L, Kagedal B, Paulsen O. Pharmacokinetics of N-acetylcysteine in man. Eur J Clin Pharmacol. 1986;31:217-22.

Pentoxifylline

Baker DE, Campbell RK. Pentoxifylline: a new agent for intermittent claudication. Drug Intell Clin Pharm. 1985;19:345-8.

Beermann B, Ings R, Mansby J, Chamberlain J, McDonald A. Kinetics of intravenous and oral pentoxifylline in healthy subjects. Clin Pharmacol Ther. 1985;37:25-8.

Ward A, Clissold SP. Pentoxifylline: a review of its pharmacodynamic and pharmacokinetic properties, and its therapeutic efficacy. Drugs. 1987;34: 50-97.

Neuromuscular Agents

Alfentanil

Van Peer A, Vercauteren M, Noorduin H, Woestenborghs R, Heykants J. Alfentanil kinetics in renal insufficiency. Eur J Clin Pharmacol. 1986;30: 245-7.

Atracurium

Conner CS. Atracurium and vecuronium: two unique neuromuscular blocking agents. Drug Intell Clin Pharm. 1984;18:714-6.

Fazadinium

Bevan DR, D'Souza J, Rouse JM, Caldwell J, Smith RL. Clinical pharmacokinetics and pharmacodynamics of fazadinium in renal failure. Eur J Clin Pharmacol. 1981;20:293-8.

Fentanyl

Mather LE. Clinical pharmacokinetics of fentanyl and its newer derivatives. Clin Pharmacokinet. 1983;8:422-46.

Gallamine

Ramzan MI, Shanks CA, Triggs EJ. Gallamine disposition in surgical patients with chronic renal failure. J Clin Pharmacol. 1981;12:141-7.

Neostigmine

Cronnelly R, Stanski DR, Miller RD, Sheiner LB, Sohn YJ. Renal function and the pharmacokinetics of neostigmine in anesthetized man. Anesthesiology. 1979;51:222-6.

Pancuronium

McLeod K, Watson MJ, Rawlings MD. Pharmacokinetics of pancuronium in patients with normal and impaired renal function. Br J Anaesth. 1976;48: 341-5.

Pyridostigmine

Cronnelly R, Stanski DR, Miller RD, Sheiner LB. Pyridostigmine kinetics with and without renal function. Clin Pharmacol Ther. 1980;28:78-81.

Succinylcholine

Bishop M, Hornbein TF. Prolonged effect of succinylcholine after neostigmine and pyridostigmine administration in patients with renal failure. Anesthesiology. 1983;58:384-6.

Sufentanil

Monk JP, Beresford R, Ward A. Sufentanil: a review of its pharmacological properties and therapeutic use. Drugs. 1988;36:286-313.

Tubocurarine

Miller RD, Matteo RS, Benet LZ, Sohn YJ. The pharmacokinetics of d-tubocurarine in man with and without renal failure. J Pharmacol Exp Ther. 1977;202:1-7.

Vecuronium

Miller RD. Vecuronium: a new nondepolarizing neuromuscular-blocking agent: clinical pharmacology, pharmacokinetics, cardiovascular effects and use in special clinical situations. Pharmacotherapy. 1984;4:238-47.

Shanks CA, Avram MJ, Fragen RJ, O'Hara DA. Pharmacokinetics and pharmacodynamics of vecuronium administered by bolus and infusion during holothane or balanced anesthesia. Clin Pharmacol Ther. 1987;42: 459-64.

Index